DESTINY FULFILLED

The Biography
of
DARRINGTON LOUIS EUGENE LOVELACE

DESTINY FULFILLED

The Biography
of
DARRINGTON LOUIS EUGENE LOVELACE

Gladys J. Seedorf, LCSW

SEEDORF BOOK PUBLISHING
Battle Creek, Michigan

DESTINY FULFILLED
The Biography of Darrington Louis Eugene Lovelace
Published by Seedorf Book Publishing
11135 Burrows Road
Battle Creek, MI 49014
(269) 968-2636
g01131963@yahoo.com

Gladys Seedorf, Publisher
Yvonne Rose, Book Packager (www.qualitypress.info)
Printed Page, Interior and Cover Design

ALL RIGHTS RESERVED

No part of this book may be reproduced or transmitted in any form or by any means – electronic or mechanical, including photocopying, recording or by any information storage and retrieved system without written permission from the authors, except for the inclusion of brief quotations in a review.

Seedorf Books are available at special discounts for bulk purchases, sales promotions, fund raising or educational purposes.

Copyright © 2016 by Gladys Seedorf
Hardcover ISBN #: 978-0-98925-90-2-6
Ebook ISBN #: 978-0-9892590-3-3
Library of Congress Control Number: 2016914568

We have one life; it soon will be past; what we do for God is all that will last.

> *Muhammad Ali, champion boxer*

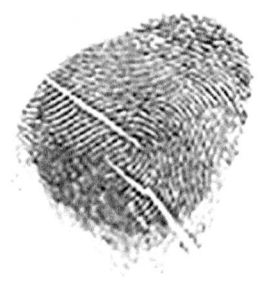 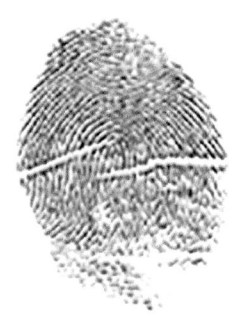

(DARRINGTON'S FINGER PRINTS)

Darrington L.E. Lovelace

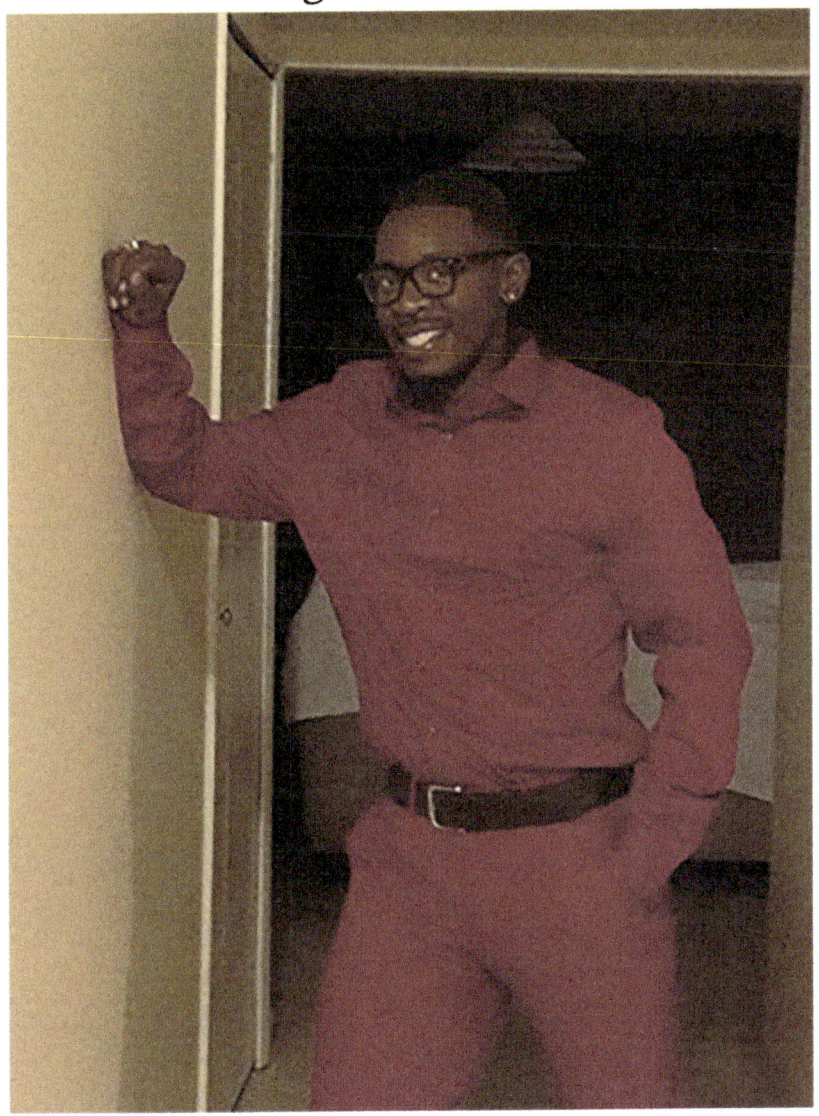

Sunrise: 2-16-1988
Sunset: 11-19-2015

DEDICATION

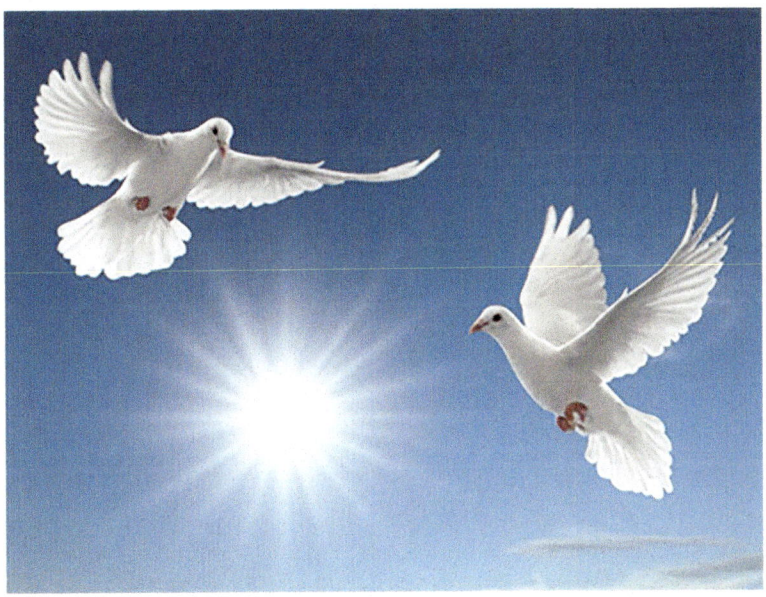

I dedicate this book to my dear sister, Lynn and her two daughters, Jaquita and Barongiere Lovelace. Please know that you will forever remain in my thoughts and prayers as you mourn the loss of such a kind and compassionate son and brother.

ACKNOWLEDGEMENTS

I give thanks and praise to the mighty risen Savior, Jesus Christ, who saw fit to once again breathe the breadth of precious life into me. My life is not for my benefit, but more, for me to be an encouragement and a blessing to others. I am merely an infinitesimal part of God's handiwork that fits into a much larger, very intricately detailed mosaic tapestry to be used as an instrument to disseminate his awe-inspiring word all over the world. My daily prayer is that my words and my actions be always lightly seasoned with salt and full of grace so that others would clearly see the love of Christ in me.

I thank my dear husband James, for being the best spouse that anyone could ever ask and for his support which I find to be truly endless. Honey from what I've seen, you're the best in the world. You are such a kind and giving person. I thank you for 31 years of marriage; but more, I pray that God would watch over you, keep you safe, healthy, and continue to shower you with his blessings all the days of your life. Perhaps it is a bit selfish of me, but I've asked God to let me enjoy you until the end of time, that's how much you mean to me my sweet love.

I send out a ginormous bouquet of yellow and white roses lightly sprinkled with Baby's Breath to my mother, Jewel Peterson. I'll never forget that you once mentioned that yellow was your favorite color. Had it not been for you and all of your hard work and efforts, I wouldn't be the person that I am today. You've been through a lot in your day, but somehow you've managed to instill in me a deep desire to genuinely care for others and more, to fear the Lord. Because of your God-given wisdom, you've taught me to treat everyone the way I would want to be treated; but more important to think for myself and not be influenced by others. I've never been one to toot my own horn, but I feel that you have done a wonderful job raising me!

I want to acknowledge my father, the late Louis Peterson with a cup of hot coffee. He too had some influence in my upbringing. Like anyone else, he had issues, but nevertheless he was the father that God assigned to me. I am also reminded that I physically resemble him and even behave like him in some ways. I guess my response to that is "Well I'll be doggoned, Louis lives on." By the way, I too love to drink a good cup of hot coffee in the morning, noon and night. I even love the smell of it.

My dear friends, Dr. Roger and Yvonne Thomson, thank you so much for being there for me when I needed someone to listen to me and for encouraging me to continue with my writing. Your support means the world to me. I mustn't forget to express my appreciation for all the nice sweet wines that you keep on hand especially for me. You know you've spoiled me rotten. Truly I consider you two as the Crème De La Crème of friends. I pray that you both would have long life and good health to enjoy each other and especially to care for all of those nice grandchildren that seem to keep coming! Truly a grandchild is a gift that keeps on giving.

George and Jeannette Martin, thanks so much for all your positive support and encouragement as well. I can always depend on you regardless of what I am planning. I feel very blessed to be acquainted with you.

Ella May Hoyt Toney, you are in a class all by yourself. I cannot think of anybody that can hold a candle to you. You are such a good and loyal friend; I seriously wouldn't trade you for all the money in the world. I mustn't forget to express my gratitude for all the nice coffee and deserts that you so graciously prepared for me over the years. I wouldn't dare neglect to offer my thanks for the beautifully embroidered gifts that you so kindly shared with me as well. Ella Mae, you are irreplaceable! Because of your genuine kindness, I pray that God will bless you and your family with his goodness and mercy which will spill over into all the generations.

Karin DeGraw, my dear friend, your friendship means the world to me. I came across a scripture that I thought perfectly described you.

> *A faithful friend is a sturdy shell. She that has found one has found a treasure. There is nothing so precious as a faithful friend, and no scales can measure her excellence. A faithful friend is an elixir of life and those who fear the Lord will find her.*
> **Sirach 6:14-16 Revised Standard Version**
> **Catholic Edition (RSVCE)**

A very special thank you goes out to two people that I once called friends, but I now refer to them as part of my immediate family, Curtis Whitaker and Scott Stokes. I've always wanted brothers and now I feel that you two are the brothers that I never had. You are the sweetest and most supportive people that I know on this side of heaven. I pray that God would continue to bless you and renew your strength so that you could mount up on wings and fly like the eagle forever.

I mustn't forget to include my dear friend Mary Jane. Thank you so much for bringing such a rare and precious jewel into my life. I feel that she too is part of my family as well.

Dr. Miriam Daly, I thank you for your genuine friendship and also for all of your many words of encouragement of my writing. "May the road rise to meet you, may the wind be always at your back, may the sun shine warm upon your face," and may God always hold you in the palm of his hand.

Tony and Yvonne Rose, Directors of Quality Press. I thank you for your wise council that you've provided me with over the years. Because of your services and expertise, I am able to share my gift of writing with the world. You have taken my manuscripts and made something absolutely beautiful of them. I have chosen to adopt you too into my family as well.

Karla Anderson, R. N, at the Turtle Dove Holistic Center. I thank you for your friendship and also your medical expertise. You gave my nephew, Darrington, hope when all others chose not to for fear of being unrealistic. He was at the lowest point in his life, yet you chose to at least give him hope, even though you knew his condition was grave. Rather than take the last skerrick of hope away, which you could have so easily done, you chose to stand by him. I will forever be grateful to you for that. Before his death he asked me to let you know how much he really appreciated you for not giving up on him. My sincere prayer for you is: long life, peace, good health, and happiness. I thank you so much.

> *Through Him we have also obtained access by faith into this grace in которой we stand, and we rejoice in hope of the glory of God.*
> **-Romans 5: 2-5**

Through Him we have also obtained access by faith into this grace in which we stand, and we rejoice in hope of the glory of God.
                                                    -Romans 5: 2-5

More than that, we rejoice in our sufferings, knowing that suffering produces endurance and endurance produces character, and character produces hope and hope does not put us to shame, because God's love has been poured into our hearts through the Holy Spirit who has been given to us.

CONTENTS

Dedication v
Acknowledgements... vii
Introduction 1

PART ONE : Darrington Louis Eugene Lovelace 11
CHAPTER ONE : The Birth... 12
CHAPTER TWO : The Middle Child 16
CHAPTER THREE : School Age 19
CHAPTER FOUR : Bowel Issues....................................... 25
CHAPTER FIVE : Limited Resources 30
CHAPTER SIX : Coming Out of the Closet 34
CHAPTER SEVEN : Like Sands Flowing
　　Through the Hourglass... 43
CHAPTER EIGHT : He Danced His Ass Off 60
CHAPTER NINE : Turtle Dove Holistic Care 67
CHAPTER TEN : Hospice House...................................... 74
CHAPTER ELEVEN : Silenced Forever 80

PART TWO: Diet & Health Research.......................... 101
CHAPTER TWELVE : Lil Bit of Wisdom 102
CHAPTER THIRTEEN : Cancer Facts............................. 104
CHAPTER FOURTEEN : Exercise 119
CHAPTER FIFTEEN : Diet & Nutrition 126
CONCLUSION 135
INDEX 141
ABOUT THE AUTHOR 143

Blessed are they that mourn; for they shall be comforted.

-Matthew 5:4

INTRODUCTION

When someone endures such a significant loss, it's very difficult to know what to say, but what I know for sure is that your son, and brother, fought with all of his mind, body, and soul to overcome the despicable Cancer. Despite having such a lengthy four-year arduous battle, we mustn't forget that God loved him enough to take him out of his pain and misery by calling him home to a land that flows with unconditional love and perfect peace. With all my heart, I believe that God not only heard our prayers but also answered them by way of the miraculous healing that we asked. There is no doubt in my mind that Darrington was healed and delivered indeed, but not in the manner that we wanted. Near the end of his life many attempts were made to revive him so that we could be blessed with his presence on this side of heaven. Somewhere in the process I believe that Jehovah allowed him to see a tiny glimpse of eternity, which greatly peaked his interests and thus enabled him to enter into a realm where nothing exists except for genuine love, peace and joy unspeakable! I'm sure that his decision was the most difficult one that he ever had to make in his life, knowing that he would leave us for a while; but surely he was consumed and securely wrapped in the arms of the precious Holy Ghost. Ah, to be wrapped in the arms of the Holy spirit which I can only compare to the newborn king being gently swaddled and cuddled by his mother, the Virgin Mary who stares right into those precious, innocent eyes. Naturally he was stupefied and I'm absolutely positive that Darrington found those split seconds that occurred within a twinkling of an eye to be totally indescribable, unlike no other comparison in the world but yet well beyond amazingly surreal. Perhaps he glimpsed loved ones that have already journeyed through this life, such as his Grandpa Louis or his Grandpa Eugene, or even his sweet Great Grandma Madeline, all in their youth of course and who all longed to share their love with him as well. I'm positive that he wanted to meet his Great Grandma Madeline, especially since he never had the pleasure of being introduced to her in this life.

As Darrington peregrinated through life, assuredly he not only realized but also accepted that he was inured a mandatory appointment with death; nor did he have the privilege of cancellation. Instead of wallowing in pity, he bore his cross like the humble and brave Christian that he was. I never once heard him say, "Why me" or "I wish I could pass this illness on to someone else" or "why not pass this illness onto some drunk homeless person." No such selfish words ever came out of his mouth. For certain his illness greatly strengthened his character, but mostly I observed that he developed a much closer and personal relationship with God.

The good shepherd loved him so much that he looked down from heaven and saw how tired his little lamb was and also the endless stream of tears that he shed at night when no one else was present. God clearly sensed fear and uncertainty in his thoughts as he was slowly being consumed by such a horrific demonic illness that only Satan himself could have unleashed. Yes, the mighty risen Savior was clearly aware that Satan camouflaged himself as an evil slithering cancer that was all too happy to invade Darrington's internal organs. The cancer prevented him from enjoying the very things in life that he loved so much. The maniacal cancer, AKA Satan, constantly roams aimlessness throughout the earth seeking whom he may devour. Since Jehovah knew that the road Darrington traveled had been extremely arduous, I believe he sent an angel to walk beside him throughout his life, but more, to tightly hold his hand while ushering him safely into heaven at the end. I cannot be sure, but I like to think that the angel was his Great Grandma Madeline who was as sweet and gentle as a lamb. Although Darrington never met her, I made it a point to speak about her on occasion, which seemed to really intrigue him.

All in all, your son and brother was sui generis and most important, he has left an amazing legacy to the world that will never be forgotten. Darrington has managed to do in 27 years what it takes some to do in a lifetime. He has mastered the three most important commandments from God: Faith, Hope and Love; the greatest of these is Love. His faith and hope in God was absolutely unquestionable. Due to his Christian upbringing he developed a close relationship with God at a very young age. It was no surprise that his faith never wavered. He put on the whole armor of God: He wore the breastplate of righteousness, loins girt with truth, feet shod with the preparation of peace, and he carried the shield of faith in his right hand; Darrington wore a helmet of salvation and held a sword of the spirit which is the word of God. Most important, he has unconditionally loved all those whose lives he touched. It seemed that no matter where he went, people seemed to be genuinely fond of him. It was so obvious that he was a Christian because he maintained such a very humble and tender demeanor. His personality perfectly represented love, kindness and compassion; and yet there was always a God- given glow that naturally shone about him. I don't know if he realized it, but his smile was very warm and contagious.

> *We know that we have passed from death to life because we love each other. Anyone that does not love remains in death.*
> **-1 John 3:14**

Even though Darrington acknowledged that his illness seemed to spiral out of control, he refused to lose hope and insisted that he would stay the course and continue to trust in the power of the almighty Jehovah Jirrah. He oft said, "I don't know what the future holds, but I will never forget who is in control of my life." I feel that he was somewhat like the character in the Bible, Job. Job was blameless, upright, feared God and shunned evil. Although God allowed the devil to take away everything that Job loved, Job still served him. The Devil was certain that Job would deny his faith especially after he maliciously attacked his health which drastically plummeted, but again Satan was a liar. Although Satan relished every minute of destroying Job's physical body, his loving family, and his vast number of cattle, he couldn't touch his soul. Even Job's wife suggested that he curse God and die; but again, Job refused and told her that she was foolish because he knew what a great and mighty God he served. I have a hunch that Job, who now sits in heaven, heard about a young man on planet earth who was also blameless, upright, God fearing and shunned evil as well. Within a split second the portals of heaven opened up and allowed him to send a supernatural message that magically traveled in and out of time, faster than the speed of light, bypassing Jupiter, Venus, Mars, Saturn, and Pluto, which burst through the atmosphere, landing precisely inside Darrington's brain becoming embedded deep within his thought processes. Wow! This information greatly encouraged him and clearly sent the message, "You too can do all things through Christ which strengthens you." Obviously Darrington received Job's message because he seemed to embrace his faith as never before; yet all the while his health continued to rapidly erode like an F 5 tornado spiraling chaotically out of control.

Now that all is said and done, I must say that I proudly stand on the sidelines and cheer for Darrington, the champion who courageously finished the race and now sits among the ranks of Job. Assuredly he will receive a jeweled crown of righteousness. Words cannot express the awesome spiritual experience that I was allowed to witness. I saw firsthand, what most people only read about. I have been deeply humbled; but more, I have been amazingly spiritually blessed and strengthened by observing the magnitude of his faith.

I want you to know that I intend to spend the rest of my life following in Darrington's footsteps in hopes of being worthy enough to one day stand before the throne of grace in the presence of the author and finisher of my faith, Jesus Christ and also your son, and brother. I will not say that he made the process look easy, but indubitably, he was under the anointing of the Holy Spirit, which allowed him to accomplish such an enormous task.

Naturally, we will lament because we miss him terribly; but we will also continue to give God all the honor, praise and glory due his name. We know that all things work together for good, for those who love God. Of course our hearts are heavy because in our opinion, Darrington's life ended much too quickly and we desperately desired just a few more seconds, minutes, hours, days. We would have settled for anything. Under no circumstances will we question God because our faith tells us that not only did He create the heavens and the earth, but that He makes no mistakes. No matter what happens we hold our heads up high, square our shoulders and walk confidently through the valley of the shadow of death and we will fear no evil because His rod and staff remain constantly with us. We venerate Him and only Him. By his stripes our sins are forgiven and we are healed. Cancer, Diabetes, HIV; nothing is too difficult for God. His name is above every name; every knee shall bow and every tongue will confess that Jesus Christ is Lord. He is puissant and worthy to be praised. Our faith also tells us that when we are absent from the body, we are present with the Lord. Because we know not how much time we have on this earth, we too must work diligently so that when God calls for us; we too will be in the presence of Darrington, Job and our Emmanuel.

As I close I leave you with few scriptures that I hold very close to my heart and I recite whenever I feel the need. It is a reminder to me that my God whom I refer to as "the big man," has my back and watches over me at all times, morning, noon, and night. Because Jesus Christ is the only one that has the power to give life and take life, I know that nothing else matters.

And I am convinced that nothing can ever separate us from God's love. Neither death nor life, neither angels nor demons, neither our fears for today nor our worries about tomorrow—not even the powers of hell can separate us from God's love. No power in the sky above or in the earth below—indeed, nothing in all creation will ever be able to separate us from the love of God that is revealed in Christ Jesus our Lord.

Romans 8:38-39 New Living Translation (NLT)

Peace I leave to you my beloved

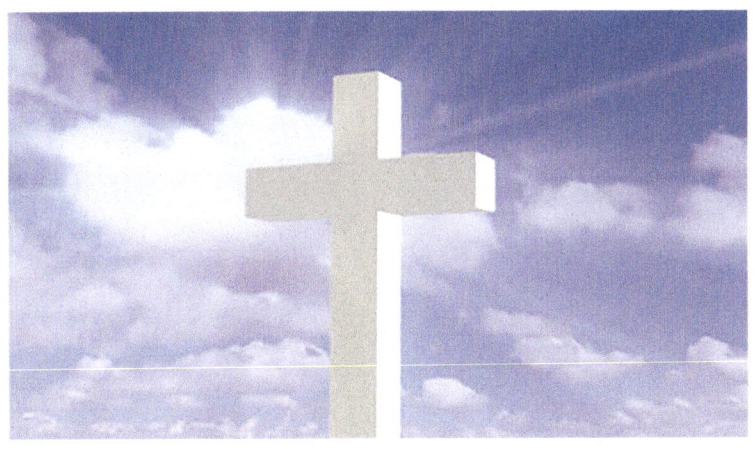

The Lord's Prayer
(Matthew 6:9-13)

Our Father in heaven,
hallowed be your name,
thy kingdom Come,
your will be done, on
Earth as it is in heaven.

Give us today our daily bread
And forgive us our debts,
as we also have forgiven our debtors.

And lead us not into temptation
but deliver us from the evil one

For thine is the Kingdom and the
power and the glory, forever and ever
Amen

PART ONE:

DARRINGTON LOUIS EUGENE LOVELACE

CHAPTER ONE

THE BIRTH

She strenuously labored for several hours in the hospital, and the nurse entered the room about every twenty to thirty minutes to evaluate the length of time between birthing pains and also to determine how fast the uterus was dilating. "You're doing just fine dear, would you like a little local anesthetic," the nurse asked. "No, I'll be fine," Lynn responded. "Okay just be sure to take deep cleansing breaths at the end of each contraction," she reminded her. "Yes of course I will," Lynn said. She was adamant that she didn't want to risk the baby receiving anything that wasn't absolutely necessary, even if it meant that she would forgo any type of assuage. Specifically, for the purpose of coaching and support during the labor and delivery process, Lynn had asked me to be present, as well as her spouse of ten years. I felt that it was truly an honor and a privilege to be asked to not only assist my sister, but also to witness the birth of my nephew. As I massaged Lynn's back, her husband, Darren sat quietly in a chair nearby. He really didn't have much to say, and was rather stoic. Finally, after a few hours Lynn was taken to the delivery room that seemed pretty frigid and actually caused my joints to stiffen. She was told that the temperature had to be kept cold for the purpose of decreasing any signs of bacteria. Because the room was so brightly lit we both felt that we might actually need our sunglasses. Fortunately, her birth pangs quickly deterred either of us from focusing on such bright lights. Finally, the doctor was summoned by the nurse and quickly arrived wearing light blue scrubs covered by a long white jacket. As he stood over to the side of the room washing his hands, he put on a mask and gloves in anticipation of delivering a baby. Two nurses stood patiently to assist as needed.

By this time the head was barely crowning and she was in full labor having very hard labor pangs. Her legs were placed in the stirrups and the doctor checked the vaginal area to determine if the head was in the crowning position. "The head is right there," said the doctor. The doctor instructed her to bear down and push as hard as she could. She pushed with all her might about five times and finally the baby was born. "Well, you have a very nice son," said the doctor as he congratulated them. "And now sir, you may cut the cord," as he handed the scissors to Darren who smiled, but was yet somewhat reserved. The doctor handed the baby to the nurse and immediately left the room.

Darren and Lynn breathed a sigh of relief as they amicably thanked the staff for their kind service. I was somewhat in shock after witnessing such an amazing process. I actually saw a real live baby work its way out of another human being. I was totally in awe. It looked as if it was quite painful but Lynn made it look so easy. I couldn't believe that she never moaned, yelled, screamed, or cried. I used to listen to the old folks at church advise the young ladies about the birthing process, "Try not to scream, because if you do, you'll lose control and besides that, you didn't scream when you was makin yo baby." I personally would have done all four in anticipation of the pain, nor would I have given two cents about those old ladies; besides, making a baby and actually having a baby are at two opposite ends of the spectrum, in my opinion. Regardless, I was so proud of my big sister for pushing her baby out like a true professional, if there was such a thing.

Although the weather was bitter cold, February 16, 1988 was a joyous occasion for Lynn and Darren as she had just given birth to a new son. After much thought and deliberation, she decided to incorporate the name of the baby's father, Darren along with both maternal and paternal Grand Fathers, Louis and Eugene to determine his name. Finally, the issue was resolved and she would call him "Darrington Louis Eugene Lovelace". At the time, Lynn and her husband were having somewhat of a rocky relationship; but nonetheless, they were the proud parents of a new bouncing baby son. At that time, the only thing that mattered was that she had delivered a healthy baby boy. His physical features resembled those of her own, which she thought was quite a nice compliment. He was awfully cute, chubby, with a hair full of black wavy curls. Assuredly, Darrington was a perfect little baby.

After about three months, Lynn noticed that Darrington was frequently fussy and not very consolable. She soon discovered that he had a little hernia. It seemed that whenever he cried, a small section of his intestines would slip down and put pressure onto his little scrotum which actually seemed to double in size. This was a very stressful time for both mama and baby. Of course, Lynn wasted no time seeking medical attention to have the hernia repaired; but, until such time occurred, she tried to keep him calm and massage his little abdomen in hopes of having the intestines return to their normal place.

She always made it a point to utilize family members who were familiar with him and would provide the care and attention that baby Darrington needed. Even though she currently had a ten-year-old daughter, Jaquita, Darrington was her first boy, her pride and joy.

Baby Darrington continued to grow and develop normally with no issues of concern. As time went on, he wasted no time crawling and finally walking as he wanted to make mischief and keep up with his big sister.

CHAPTER TWO
THE MIDDLE CHILD

Altogether, Darrington had two siblings. His oldest sister, Jaquita who is actually ten years older and a younger sister, Barongiere is two years younger than he. Though Darrington loved both his sisters, he obviously developed a closer relationship with his younger sister, most likely because they are so close in age. Because he was the middle child, there were times that he felt ignored, which is common, and nothing unusual in my opinion.

His mother worked full time as a Phlebotomist while taking college classes; his father worked sporadically but most often chose to spend more time with friends or participate in recreational activities rather than his immediate family. Nevertheless, both were preoccupied with their own lives.

Unfortunately, Darrington never developed a positive relationship with his father, or any other male figure for that matter, until he grew up. He was too young to realize that his mother struggled to put food on the table and make ends meet while trying to hold her marriage and the family together. He was too young to know that his maternal grandparents often provided financial support to his mother to help with rent, groceries, utilities; nor was he old enough to remember that his parents separated with no plans to reunite.

Eventually, the time came when his mother reluctantly took him and his two sisters to move in and live with our parents indefinitely. Although his grandmother, Jewel, was very loving and kind, his grandfather, Louis was verbally and physically abusive and his moods seemed to fluctuate at a whim. Based on today's standards, he would be diagnosed as having severe Bipolar Disorder.

I would describe Darrington's childhood as quite an emotional roller coaster that frequently ebbed and flowed from one end of the spectrum to the other. His opinion of his father was that of neglect, which often left him feeling very alone, confused and ignored; but on the other hand, his grandfather Louis was extremely temperamental. One minute he could be as gentle as a lamb and the next minute he could be as explosive as a landmine that went off without warning. It was really quite a dilemma for such a young lad to deal with.

Shortly after Lynn and her children moved in with her parents, Darrington developed a bit of a problem with his speech. I suspect that his stuttering behavior was most likely due to anxiety, as a result of being in a new, but also a very volatile and abusive environment. I witnessed Darrington be lambasted by his grandfather on many occasions. Unfortunately, no one in the house was exempt from the abuse. The onset of the stuttering seemed to ensue rather quickly, and lasted for at least six or seven months before coincidentally disappearing.

Regrettably there were no other options or living arrangements available at the time and Lynn knew that she needed a place to live that was rent free in order to spend what little money she had towards the cost of college. At one time, she aspired to go to medical school, but because life has a way of taking us on its journey, she later aspired to become a Registered Nurse, which was more realistic based on her current circumstances. It was obvious that she had no choice but to pull herself up by her bootstraps and support her three children. As time went on she continued to work full time, in addition to struggling with college classes, which meant she too had even less time to spend with any of her children. It was unfortunate, but her children would just have to learn to stay out of grandpa's way just as she had done as a child. However, she worked as hard as she could to get herself and her children out of such a less than ideal situation.

Lynn was well aware of the fact that she had brought her three children into an extremely dysfunctional environment, but she could only hope and pray that it would be temporary. Although her parents were very reliable babysitters, she often had a rough time trying to have peace of mind, considering our Bipolar father who was downright hard to live with and very unreasonable. There were many times that she felt as though she and the children had jumped from a burning fire into the flame. She too felt as though she was caught between a rock and a hard spot with no option of getting out. After almost two years, she finally graduated with an RN (Registered Nurse) degree and, needless to say, she moved out into her own apartment very shortly thereafter.

CHAPTER THREE

SCHOOL AGE

Darrington attended the Albion Public Schools. By this time, he was in Middle School and then on to High School, which certainly brought some relief and happy times. He certainly didn't need a babysitter and or rides to or from school. Finally, he could get out from under the boot of his Grandpa Louis, which had definitely affected his self-esteem. By this time, he was older, more independent and able to fend for himself, and just a delightfully fun person to be around. By the grace of God, he had managed to maintain a wonderful bonhomie personality. As he spread his wings his mother discovered that he was extremely social and very talented, as well.

Darrington became involved in lots of after school activities that were of particular interest to him. He became engrossed in: local 4H activities, sewing, singing and dancing, which were all very time consuming, but also fun and relaxing for him. Because Albion was such a small town, he practically knew everyone that lived there. He had no trouble finding rides to activities and if he did, he could walk practically wherever he wanted to go. He even tried his hand at wrestling and the swim team, which he later decided that neither were his forte.

It was no surprise that he was interested in sewing, because both his mother and grandmother were excellent seamstresses. Darrington would spend hours watching them create beautiful garments. He too was able to make a few garments that were almost as nice. Surprisingly he had a lot of patience and persistence that most young boys don't have. Because he possessed these two important attributes Darrington eventually became a very good seamstress. At one time, his mother thought he would consider going to college to be a Fashion Designer.

She realized that he was a born leader and definitely not a follower, even at such a young age. She was proud of him for not being negatively influenced by others; but instead, he carved out his own path. He opted to join the National Association for the Advancement of Colored People in order to keep abreast of current political events, locally and globally. He quickly noticed the fact that minorities were not always judged on the basis of their character, but instead, on the color of their skin. Of course Darrington never used his race as a crutch; he often saw his mother and his grandparents work hard; and he was determined to follow in their footsteps.

It was of no surprise that Darrington always put a lot of emphasis on his appearance. When he went to school he wanted to wear really stylish clothes, as often as possible. He would stand in front of the mirror and primp until he felt satisfied; after all he had to make a good impression on the young ladies, as well. His hygiene and his hair style was of the utmost importance and he made it a point to have his hair cut regularly to represent the current style at the High School. Regardless of how limited his mother's income, she always tried to buy the styles of clothing that she knew he liked. Of course the sale racks were very familiar to her as well. He was known at the high school for being one of the best dressers.

I will praise the LORD all my life; I will sing praise to my God as long as I live.

Psalm 146:2

As a young child Darrington was a member of the Battle Creek Boys Choir that met weekly and consisted of about 25-30 young boys. Darrington absolutely loved to sing and perform in front of any audience. I guess he felt that he was somewhat of a professional, especially since he was required to travel and fellowship with the other members of the choir. It was really a good match for him and his personality, as well. As a matter of fact, he was very disappointed when he was finally told that the tone of his voice changed and that he should segue into the adult male chorus.

Darrington was raised in the church and loved to sing in the choir and also participate in the Praise and Worship service. Since he previously lived with his granny as a small child, she made sure that he developed a close relationship with God by observing her praying and singing. A good hand clappin, toe tappin inspirational gospel song was an excellent precursor to a spirit-filled sermon, which most always resulted in Darrington parading around the church boldly thanking and praising God. This was what he frequently observed among the members of the church, so in turn he was strongly encouraged to worship and make a joyful noise unto the Lord, as well.

On occasion, he chose to attend and visit other churches and while doing so he experienced that some religions were just the opposite and were extremely reserved and they preferred to worship God in a much quieter way. He was taught that his faith and belief in God was no better than any other; but instead, he believed in making a joyful noise when praising God. As a result, Darrington respected, learned and developed an appreciation for many religions.

A time to laugh; and a time to dance
Ecclesiastics 3:4

Darrington absolutely loved to dance to a good Bee Bop Hip Hop song or just any good rhythmic song. The more strenuous, the better he loved it and never broke a sweat. His amateur dancing really seemed to pave the way for the professional dance that followed. I would describe Darrington's dancing as that of a youthful butterfly that had just come out of its cocoon. He was young, vibrant, and full of infinite energy.

Ballroom and Mime dancing were definitely his favorite and he made both look so easy; and his moves were smoother than a baby's bottom. Of course, the fact that he was tall, dark, and handsome didn't hurt a bit either. When he danced and began to do the movements, it was awesome to watch. Dancing allowed him to use his imagination to escape and do and be wherever and whoever he wanted to be. When he danced, he had no problems, didn't need anything, he just loved every minute of it. He was truly free! Really, it seemed that he literally somehow became a part of the song. At his church, Faith Temple Word of Faith Ministries; he performed spiritual dances to his favorite songs and it would either make you cry tears of joy or you would get up and start dancing and swaying to the music. Rhythm was his middle name. That's my nephew!

His advanced dancing skills also enabled him to choreograph the movements without any training and; without a doubt, he was definitely a force to be reckoned with. "Spiritual Beginnings," was the name of the dance ministry that Darrington and his sister Barongiere cofounded. Though they had not performed in years, their dance routines remain etched in the minds of many.

Some people find it helpful to take dancing lessons, while others have a God-given talent. The latter was true of Darrington and he could have easily studied Terpsichorean subjects at the School of Dance, Julliard in New York if he wanted to. Although some were curious, but it was never determined from which parent he received his dancing abilities because neither could ever hold a candle to him. His younger sister would often perform dance routines with him and her style was quite prepossessing, but his was absolutely stellar. An old familiar French term perfectly describes his style of dancing and is referred to as, "Joie de vivre," which means to delight in being alive, carefree. Darrington lived his life through his dancing.

Wisdom is the principal thing; therefore, get wisdom: and with all thy getting get understanding.
Proverbs 4: King James Version (KJV)

In addition to all of the wonderfully impressive twirling and swirling, Darrington was also remarkably academically talented. Not only did he want to look as though he knew what he was doing, he actually wanted to be able to speak and write intelligently. He spent a lot of time with his granny who wasn't the least bit bashful about her desire for him to attend college, "I don't want no dummies in the family," she said. "Unless them doctors done tol you, you got some kind of problem, then you beta to go on to college" she insisted that everyone in the family should go to college and get some type of higher education via degree or certificate. She felt that if she could go back to school at the age of 65 to obtain a GED with all of her health problems, then the younger generation had no excuse, nor was she about to accept any excuses. Darrington highly respected his granny and he set out to do exactly what she and his mother instructed him to do.

Though he wasn't sure which subjects he was most interested in he took all his class work very seriously and of course was a member of the National Honor Society. Obviously, he was well- liked by all of his instructors; and on the other hand, he was very respectful to his instructors. Because he was such a true gentleman, Darrington had a reputation of being "every teacher's dream." Unsurprisingly, most all of his high school instructors attended his Graduation Open House.

CHAPTER FOUR

BOWEL ISSUES

In spite of all the fun and excitement that the Middle and High Schools brought, there were some physical issues that were not so nice and quite bothersome to him for many years. It seemed that Darrington was plagued with bouts of constipation, as well as an occasional fainting spell.

Since constipation and bowel irregularity definitely weren't the coolest topic for teenagers to discuss, he kept that unfortunate part of his life close to the vest. If you had any intention of attracting a girlfriend, you certainly couldn't be walking around farting and or passing out, regardless of how good looking you thought you were. Besides that, nobody wants to be your friend if you were in the habit of passing gas. If the boys are farting, the girls insist that you've either got yourself a case of the cooties and or you're made of snakes and snails and puppy dog tails. By this time, the teachers had most likely lost control of the classroom because everybody was laughing and covering their noses. Normally, the student would be ordered out of the classroom while she emptied an entire can of air freshener into the environment, in hopes of regaining control; but sometimes that only made it worse. During that era, there wasn't as much focus on diet, fruits and vegetables, acidic as opposed to alkaline, organic and or non-organic, MSG, processed as opposed to natural foods.

Like most, Darrington came from a family that struggled to make ends meet and since most growing boys are known for inhaling instead of chewing their foods, his diet nor his digestion process weren't always the greatest. His mother and grandmother certainly did the best they could to prepare home cooked meals; but in Darrington's opinion, McDonalds restaurant, Burger King, pizza, milk shakes sounded pretty good too. During High School, he worked at McDonalds; and I'm sure he had his share of Big Macs, heavily salted fries with lots of extra ketchup, and a big sugary Coke product, as well. Water, which is now known as the miracle drug was never emphasized to Darrington because it was a different time.

Regardless of how friendly, and or talented he was there was little attention paid to such a very essential issue. Regardless, he somehow managed to grow up and move along just fine, even though he was a quite constipated at times. Nevertheless, he was young, strong and felt as though the sky was the limit.

High school was over and It was now time for college. At the age of eighteen, Darrington proudly headed off to Michigan State University to study. He had not yet declared an area of study as he wasn't exactly sure what he wanted to focus on, which is pretty common for most Freshman. Who cares what they study as long as they get their general studies out of the way, which are a requirement as well. Naturally, Darrington really seemed to enjoy being away from home, away from the supervision of his mother and grandparents, etc.

Shortly into the semester, all of a sudden he experienced severe abdominal pain. Once again, he seemed to be plagued with the same irritable bowel issues and fainting spells. By this time, his mother, a nurse, became very concerned about the nature of his health problems. On several occasions, she would drive up to the college to get him, to take him to the doctor to be evaluated. At that time, it was never really determined what was causing his problems. It was very frustrating for Darrington as he was trying to enjoy what was supposed to be the best four years of his life. After his first year, his mother advised him to transfer to a school closer to home so that she could keep a closer eye on him. Well, this certainly wasn't the ideal situation for him and quite frankly it was a big disappointment, but as usual he obliged.

Darrington later transferred to Albion College, which was nice; but he quickly formed a rather negative opinion. For starters, he didn't like being so close to home. He had a roommate that was also from Albion, but he felt that he didn't really have the opportunity to get to know him because their schedules were very different. As usual, there were always financial issues to address, that seemed never ending. Although he received a scholarship, there was still the issue of mandatory parental financial assistance.

Although his mother was a Registered Nurse, she had her hands full trying to manage all of the household utilities in addition to covering at least a portion of the cost towards his college. All in all, he just felt that it wasn't a good fit, so he decided to chuck the Albion College experience and find a job in order to save money for a school that he really wanted to attend, especially since his medical condition seemed to be overshadowing his life. At the time, he felt that his current situation was no more than a hiccup and that his situation would improve as time went on.

Because of Darrington's deep seeded academic ambitions, he desperately wanted to return to college not only to make his parents proud, but more, to have a better life and worry less about daily financial stressors. He struggled financially, but that was nothing unusual. "Anything that comes too easy isn't worth having," I reminded him. He and his siblings mentioned that perhaps they would one day open their own Home Care Agency. His eldest sister, Jaquita, previously graduated with a degree in Occupational Therapy, and his youngest sister said she intended to study Speech Therapy when her time came.

Alas, a year or so had gone by and his medical condition was at least fairly stable. He was sick of the rat race and was determined to go back to college and finally get his life together. He applied and was accepted into the Henry Ford Community College in Dearborn, Michigan, which he dearly loved; and of course he excelled academically. He had finally found his niche. He was an extraordinary student with definite plans to complete his Associates Degree and then transfer to Wayne State University to obtain his Bachelor's Degree in Physical Therapy before doing great and awesome things in the world. He was off to a good start, sort of like a Race Horse being let out of the stable.

Once again, his health began to teeter totter and would eventually force him to drop out of college for at least a semester. Because all the classes in the program were scheduled, he had to wait until they were being offered again, which were a real waste of time to him. Of course he was greatly disappointed, but he knew he had been ill and there was realistically no way to catch up. Another semester came around and his health improved just enough to get his hopes up again, so he went back for the second time. This time he was like a gigantic Steam Roller and was truly ready to rock and roll, ready to kick butt.

Consequently, after a short time, his illness caught up with him again, like a thief in the knight. Before he knew it, the symptoms came back with a vengeance. He had no choice except to drop out of school again. He felt so downtrodden and disappointed. "All I want to do is go to school," he said. "I know," said his mother, "but let's save your life first, you have your whole life ahead of you." Of course he was very disappointed with his harrowing medical condition.

By this time his professors were losing patience and strongly encouraged him to withdraw from his studies until his health improved, which was also very hurtful. He mentioned that one of his instructors went so far as to tell him that he wasn't going to survive and that he should go ahead and withdraw from the college. Deep down, he knew the instructors were being realistic, but he just wasn't ready to roll over and play dead, just to satisfy them. He had such high hopes, that his illness would improve and he was going to hang onto his faith, no matter what. I think we've all been there at one time or another. Once again the air in his academic balloon was slowly deflating.

CHAPTER FIVE
LIMITED RESOURCES

The next year was even more stressful for Darrington as his income plummeted. It was very difficult to find a decent job, especially with no type of formal education. As a last resort, he was able to find part-time employment at a clothing store. His health wasn't the greatest, his car was on its last leg and he desperately needed reliable transportation. He found a used car, but he still needed some financial assistance from his mother. Needless to say, Darrington was frustrated with his situation, but he never gave up and always tried to forge ahead. His long term goals never changed and he still aspired to graduate from college.

Unfortunately, he was not able to save much money, especially since he was only earning minimum wage which had to cover his living expenses. Because money was so scarce, he was forced to make poor food choices, which is pretty common when there is an abundance of bills and very little money to work with. Despite the fact that his journey through life seemed to only go one way, he was determined to press on and maintain a positive attitude, hoping that things would someday change. His mother helped out as much as she could, but she too had her hands full.

Sadly, Darrington's father was seldom involved in his life long enough to offer any kind of moral or financial support. Occasionally he could recall when his father took him and his sisters to visit relatives, but there was nothing constant about his presence, or the role that he played in his life. Darrington said he had no recollection of his father taking him to the park to play ball, or to a movie, or just to sit and watch television. As a child he could recall no regular visitations and minimal to no child support being provided, etc.

Regrettably, coming into his adult stage was no different as far as Darrington was concerned. He had no explanation of why he received no paternal support, nor did he try to make any excuses for his father. He clearly knew his father, and even saw him occasionally, but there was no genuine love loss. Darrington often appeared to be rather hurt and confused, but he tried not to dwell on it, nor did he ever confront his father. Darrington was indeed a master of concealing his feelings. Although he spoke very little about his father, he never indulged in making negative comments; instead, he maintained a certain line of respect for him. Typically, his comments went no further than, "I just don't know." It was obvious that he never stopped loving him, regardless of their limited contact.

Darrington knew he could always count on his mother and the immediate family. We were his rock. No matter what happened in his life, we all tried to be there to protect, provide support, encourage, provide financial assistance, etc. Although we did our best to be there for Darrington, it was obvious that we too were sometimes spread thin and overwhelmed.

Although I lived a short distance away, he knew he could count on me as well for financial support and encouragement. Although he never asked me for money, I wouldn't hesitate to offer, especially if I had the available funds. Darrington was always very respectful and gracious towards me whenever he received any kind of assistance. His humble and appreciative attitude really made me want to give him more, which is most of what happened. I dearly loved him as though he was my own son and he loved me as well. We had a special bond between us that neither of us would ever forget.

Darrington loved to visit me because I lived in the country. He really enjoyed the quiet as there wasn't much traffic going down my road. In the summer, he enjoyed the grapes from the grapevines, he loved to swim in the pool, or just sit on the deck and enjoy watching the chickens. Heck, he even said he loved to ride in my GMC Acadia truck. I think he liked it because it was big and so was he. He had plenty of room to lean back and relax. He typically wanted the heater and the seat warmers to be set as high as possible because he was always cold. Unfortunately, I just happened to be going through my change of life and was having severe hot flashes. By the time we reached our destination, I was usually dripping wet with sweat. Regardless, I turned the heat up as high as Darrington wanted it, which really didn't bother me.

He loved the Sirius XM radio as it gave him the opportunity to scroll the stations and find his favorite Gospel Artists. Once he found it, he turned the volume up really loud so that he could clearly hear the sound of the Bose Base. We both sat and bobbed our heads up and down, swaying back and forth to the sound of the music. I'm sure that the other drivers thought we were jammin to the latest Rhythm and Blues song, but we loved many of the same Christian artists. One of his favorites in particular was a song entitled -

"My Words Have Power," by Karen Clark Sheard and Donald Lawrence.

Sometimes I felt like the whole truck was rocking to the beat and often wondered if the truck was even touching the ground, but I never said a word as I wanted him to be comfortable and besides, he was my big Teddy Bear. As if that wasn't enough, I catered to him even more by preparing foods that he liked, but yet were good for him. All in all, I spoiled him rotten and we both really loved it! I've learned that you just can't be too nice to anyone.

CHAPTER SIX

COMING OUT OF THE CLOSET

At some point in Darrington's life, he decided to "come out of the closet" and declare that he was gay. He never said how long he had been having those feelings, but in hindsight, we did recall that he didn't seem to have any special female friends that he dated and or regularly brought home. I guess he wanted to spend time with everybody. Quite frankly for any member of the family to announce that he or she was involved in a homosexual relationship was appalling, at least initially.

The historical teachings of the church were very matter of fact and against those types of relationships…one man, one woman and absolutely forbid any of the members to indulge themselves especially if they had any desire of going to heaven to be with the risen Savior and take that wonderful ride in one of those awesome chariots. Of course, the news took the members of our family by surprise as nobody understood his decision, nor did he ever offer any explanation, most likely because he was of age. On the flip side of that coin, perhaps he too had lots of questions about his childhood and the dysfunctional behaviors that occurred in the family, which were never explained to him as well.

Certainly his mother had all the normal feelings that most parents have. She was very frustrated, disappointed, but yet somewhat afraid. She knew that her son didn't need her permission, but, this was probably the first time in her life that she really wished he needed her approval. Although she never said, but I'm sure her thoughts were running a mile a minute. What will people say? What will they think? How will I explain it or perhaps I can just pretend that I know nothing about it? It certainly wasn't uncommon to hear or read that LGBT's have been treated unfairly and or have been victims of hate crimes. She knew that he had entered into a realm where she wouldn't be able to protect him that left her feeling helpless, confused, embarrassed, etc. Nevertheless, Darrington wasn't asking for anybody's permission at this stage, just their unconditional love which he felt he was entitled to.

Basically Darrington's relationship with his partner was no different from any other heterosexual relationship. There were good and bad days, on and off days, but all in all it was his decision that we had to live with. By no means were we going to disown him or withhold our love and affection.

Unfortunately, Lynn's feelings toward his partner was somewhat of a different story. She held sort of a neutral negative opinion of him. I never heard Darrington speak of him, at least in the presence of his mother; nor did he ever invite him to celebrate any of the holidays with the family. He and I spoke of him occasionally. Perhaps the feelings towards his partner may have been different had Darrington presented a different picture of him, I cannot say for sure. For certain, his partner was very involved in his care at least as much as possible. There were times when Darrington sought just as much support from his partner as the immediate family and he spent quite a bit of time with him as well, especially earlier on in his illness.

Coincidentally, I just happened to run into his partner during one of Darrington's many hospital stays. He very comfortably introduced his partner who I found to be very cordial and pleasant. My first impression of him was that of surprise. He was tall, slim, fair skinned, neatly dressed and, in my opinion, real good-looking. What stood out most was the fact that he had the most beautifully manicured nails with bright orange nail polish and a matching hand bag that hung over his shoulder. After looking at him for a few seconds, I kind of felt that perhaps I should have put more emphasis into my own appearance before I left home; but I quickly moved beyond that point. I grabbed my purse from a nearby chair, tossed it onto the floor and motioned for him to sit down next to me. He smiled and immediately picked my purse up off the floor and said, "Oh no honey, we don't throw our bags on the floor." He gently laid my purse at the foot of the bed where Darrington lay. He and I warmly embraced and enjoyed each other's company.

On several occasions his partner mentioned how nice I smelled and how I reminded him of one of his favorite aunts. It was really quite a warm, mutually respectful and non-judgmental conversation, which definitely seemed to put Darrington's mind at ease. I would have loved to have had them over for dinner had Darrington not been required to spend so much time in the hospital.

Regardless of anybody's sexual orientation, I felt it was not my place to pass judgement. I always made it a point to try to live by the words of the Holy Bible that clearly states that God will judge everyone according to his or her deeds and also that everyone should love thy neighbor as themselves, which includes everybody: Thy Homeless Neighbor, Thy Muslim Neighbor, Thy Black Neighbor, Thy Gay Neighbor, Thy White Neighbor, Thy Jewish Neighbor, Thy Christian Neighbor, Thy Atheist Neighbor, Thy Racist Neighbor, Thy Alcohol and Drug Addicted Neighbor, Thy Mentally illness Neighbor and or Physically Handicapped Neighbor. I thought this was superb and quite frankly it took a big load off my list of things to do since I realized that I didn't have to judge how others choose to live their lives. Fortunately, it gave me more time to focus on more pleasant things. I felt that by the time I genuinely loved others and treated them as I wanted to be treated, then the day would be over.

I specifically raised my children to respect all people and to treat them as they too would want to be treated. A mere learned behavior from my Mama who said, "Dont neva forget dat everybody have feelins and everybody want to be treated nice." To dismiss someone because of their sexual orientation is ludicrous and neither I nor my immediate family members intend to miss out on any part of life because of it. Some of my dearest friends are gay and or lesbian, and I love them just as much or more than those that aren't.

As a matter of fact, I definitely feel that the LGBTQ population is definitely unfeigned as opposed to many Christians that claim to be totally free from sin, sanctified, and filled with his precious holy ghost. I guess I remain confused by the "True and Super Christians" that regularly indulge in extra marital affairs while others don't even care to keep things secret. Some have been caught embezzling money from large corporations where they've been employed for years, and even some of our elected officials continue to make poor political decisions that clearly negatively impact the elderly, poor, and helpless children, who are the least able to defend themselves while the wealthy remain unscathed. Some "True and Super Christians" just think they're downright better than others simply because they show up at church on Sunday and write out a big Fat Cat check and or because they've inherited millions and now the world suddenly needs to bow down to them. Some have had opportunities made available to them where others have not, which is a blessing in my opinion; but it is certainly not an entitlement to treat others as if they don't meet their standards.

I feel that some, not all "True and Super Christians" are racists and or bigots. Oh here's another one to mull over. What about all the Pastors and Evangelists that think they're so high and mighty and feel they're entitled to date many women in the church, meanwhile they summon all "sinners" of the congregation to quickly get in the prayer line to pray for forgiveness. I'm so sick and tired of hearing Pastors stand up in front of the congregation and say, "God told me to do this or that which we know couldn't possibly be true. I like what my Mama said, "God aint tol you nothin, and you just sittin up there lyin yo tale off." My question is…"Are we really supposed to look the other way and label these people as True and Super Christians?

Do we honestly think these so called "True and Super Christians" will be found in heaven sitting at the banquet table communing with my redeemer, the Prince of Peace while the entire LGBTQ population is condemned to spend eternity in a lake of fire gnashing their teeth?

> ***But God made the earth by his might; he shaped the world by his wisdom, crafted the skies by his knowledge.***
>
> **- Jeremiah 10:12**

For those of us who definitely don't want to miss the "Heaven Exit," it would behoove all of us who live in this sin sick world to quietly focus on our own imperfections, rather than waste precious time addressing the sexual orientation of others, especially since God has clearly indicated that HE would do the judging. Surely if He created the heavens, the earth and everything therein; I don't have the foggiest notion how I or anyone else could possibly feel qualified and or be of any help to judge the LGBTQ's, bigots, pastors, murderers, lazy liars, full bodied tattooed, morbidly obese individuals, etc.

In the words of Reverend James Cleveland, we better "Get right church and let's go home." Assuredly, we would do better to stop Policing the lifestyle of others and be more aware of our own shortcomings for fear that we may actually be the ones to end up in the lake of fire. Since we know that the coming of the Lord will occur as fast as a twinkling of an eye and or a thief in the night, then we really have no spare time to dilly dally around, in my opinion.

I feel that our society forgets that the LGBTQ don't ask to be born, nor do they ask to have the emotions, feelings, that they have. I don't believe that anybody gets up in the morning and says, "Oh gee, I've got nothing else to do, perhaps I'll be Transgender today." Based on my research, Epigenetics play a huge role in the behavior of the genes of all individuals.

Epigenetics effect how our genes express themselves and are determined by the environment in which we live, and as a result are passed onto our offspring. Genes respond to accurate life-affirming perceptions and also to misperceptions. Consequently, the nature of our perceptions greatly influence the fate of our lives.

Undoubtedly there is scientific data that offers explanation regarding LGBTQ, just as there is any other health and human condition. Rather than try to annihilate the LGBTQ population, why don't we act like the True and Super Christians that we say we are and at least offer some support and at least make some appropriate referrals where help can be obtained. I am reminded of the awesome and famous Basketball player, Magic Johnson who shocked the nation in 1991 when he announced that he had been diagnosed with HIV that often dispels the stigma of being gay. Until he came forth the HIV population was shunned and black-balled in my opinion. Following his announcement, all types of money and support were suddenly poured into his diagnosis for the purpose of research.

The Howard Brown Health Center, named after Dr. Howard Brown, is located in Chicago, Illinois and is the nation's largest organization that services the LGBTQ population. This health center provides cutting edge, trend specific treatment that addresses many issues, provides medications, counseling, surgery, to make the individual more comfortable and able to manage specific issues and or concerns.

I am very thankful that this organization exists. I fear that those who continue to be indifferent towards the LGBTQ population will one day wake up and find that their own children, grandchildren and or great grandchildren will announce that he or she is LGBTQ; perhaps then, kindness, understanding and compassion will be received. Finally, it will be understood that neither being African American and or LGBTQ is transmitted by a handshake, hug or even a kiss.

In the words of Robin Williams, *"We all have issues, let's just be kind to each other, let's not waste time pointing out our differences."*

Pastor Elmer Hess said, "Now don't y'all fool yourselves, EVERYBODY AINT going to heaven and when you finally get to heaven, you will have three surprises: 1) you will notice that those you were sure would be present will actually be unfound 2) you will notice that those who you were certain would be absent, will be clearly visible and 3) the fact that you actually made it, will be pretty amazing." Pastor said a lot of good things, but for some reason those words remain etched in my mind.

I have recently joined the Battle Creek Pride organization which supports the LGBTQ population. My reasons for doing so were not because I want to encourage people to come out of the closet and announce their sexual orientation as LBGTQ; but instead I feel that everyone deserves to be treated equal which certainly includes LGBTQ. I intend to do whatever I can to support their efforts, just as I would assist any other organization that I belong to. I am a proud ally, but more, I'm proud because both my parents raised me to think this way, regardless of what anyone else feels. Neither of my folks was highly educated nor did it ever seem that they had adequate funds, but at least they had sense enough to treat others as they themselves wanted to be treated. In my opinion their actions represent "True and Super Christianity."

"If you judge people, you have no time to love them."

— **Mother Teresa**

"I have friends who are gay and we study the Bible together."

-Prince Rogers Nelson

Thank you for making me so wonderfully complex! Your workmanship is marvelous--how well I know it.

Psalm 139:14 New Living Translation

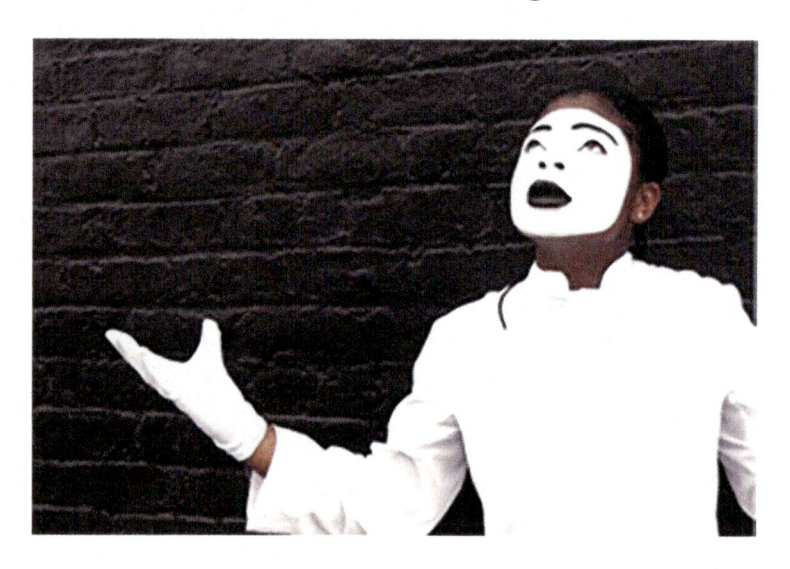

CHAPTER SEVEN

LIKE SANDS FLOWING THROUGH THE HOURGLASS

By this time, Darrington was 24-years-old. It seemed as though he had endured nothing but a lifetime of abdominal discomfort and bowel issues that were quite bothersome. Unfortunately, this time was something new and unlike any other pain he had felt in the past. The pain that he now experienced was more constant, severe and showed no signs of cessation. Not only did he experience significant pain in the abdominal region, but in his lower back, as well. Neither he nor his mother felt that it was anything serious, as he had experienced similar symptoms in the past, except this time the pain seemed a bit more severe. *Perhaps it was just a stubborn case of constipation that had reared its ugly head once again*, Darrington wondered.

Nonetheless, he remained in the hospital for about two weeks as the doctors had great difficulty diagnosing his illness. Of course his mother was concerned, but she thought the doctors would simply run the usual tests, do some blood work, prescribe some medications and send him on his merry little way. As time went on, it seemed that neither of the doctors were able to provide a concrete diagnosis.

Naturally everyone's level of anxiety rose, but nobody said a word. Darrington really didn't seem to mind being in the hospital; after all he was being given adequate pain medicine intravenously which made him very comfortable and was definitely better than he would have felt at home. "Could it possibly be Crohn's disease?" Lynn suggested to the doctors. She reported that one his cousins, Monique had spent the last few years battling that ungodly disease that nearly claimed her life. Though the possibility of Crohn's disease was presented to the doctors as a hereditary illness; it was quickly ruled out just as fast as it was mentioned. It seemed that the only response the doctors would give was, "He is very sick," which was pretty apparent based on his pain level. Regardless, everyone tried to be patient and polite without becoming too anxious. Throughout Darrington's hospitalization he received the nicest cards and a few plants, which definitely lifted his spirits. The cards read: Get Well Soon, hope you have a speedy recovery, trust in the Lord with all thine heart. Because he had such a long history with abdominal intestinal issues, nobody really knew what to expect, we all just continued to pray the prayers of faith. Darrington's grandmother, Jewel, whom he referred to as, "Granny," was a known prayer warrior and strongly believed in anointing the body with blessed oil while calling down fire from heaven. This was very comforting to Darrington who always welcomed her prayers, after all, he felt that she was somehow directly connected to God's supernatural main line to Heaven and if anybody could get a prayer through, it was his granny. Each time she went to visit she insisted on praying before she left. When she prayed, whomever was in the room would join hands while encircling Darrington. United in faith, we proceeded to boldly approach the throne of grace with prayers and with the faith of a mustard seed that Darrington was going to be just fine.

Furthermore, everyone comfortably quoted another very familiar passage of scripture from Matthew 18:19

> *Again I say unto you, That if two of you shall agree on earth as touching any thing that they shall ask, it shall be done for them of my Father which is in heaven.*

Obviously Darrington was from a family of very devout Christians, that hung on to every word of God. Because they had such a strong Christian belief, it made the whole ordeal much easier to cope with. The fact that medical staff were coming and going in and out of the room while we prayed and praised God didn't faze us one bit. We went right on with our chants and prayers while the medical staff were very respectful to us. There were times that they too joined in, as well.

Initially, Darrington had been young enough to be on his mother's medical insurance, but since he was rapidly approaching the magical age of twenty-seven he applied for Social Security Disability benefits. Because of the nature of his illness, he was immediately granted financial benefits. It was also determined that he was also eligible for Medicaid insurance benefits as a secondary payer. Because he didn't have much of a work history, his Social Security Disability Insurance was quite minimal, but at least he had something to call his own.

Almost three weeks had gone by since Darrington had finally received medical information that his diagnosis was Stage Four Colon Cancer, which meant that not only was the Colon, but also the Lymph nodes were under attack. To add insult to injury, he was also told that his type of cancer was hereditary. My perception of what I heard was *death sentence*, I thought to myself. The Oncologist suggested that immediate surgery be performed. Of course the news took everyone by surprise, but the family decided early on that they would band together and beat the illness; after all, his mother was a very seasoned Registered Nurse and she certainly had excellent relationships with many of the Oncology doctors, and she felt that she knew the right questions to ask.

Darrington knew from the very beginning that he had been given quite a peril diagnosis and that it was going to be a rough and treacherous uphill road. He felt that his strength and youth were to his advantage and he was ready for the challenge. After all, he was taught to believe in miraculous healings as were performed by Jesus in the Bible. He tried hard not to dwell on it, but naturally he felt as though a rug had just been snatched from underneath him. He had also spoken with each of his doctors who indicated that it was really important to keep a positive outlook. A few days before surgery was scheduled, Darrington made sure that he informed a few close friends and family of his diagnosis as he felt that everyone could ban together and send up prayers, which is exactly what we did:

> ***If my people who are called by my name humble themselves and pray and seek my face and turn from their wicked ways, then I will hear from heaven and will forgive their sin and heal their land.***
>
> **2 Chronicles 7:14.**

The day of the surgery, Darrington's family met at the hospital. Obviously he and everyone else were terribly anxious and couldn't wait for the day's end. The surgeon came in and introduced himself and informed everyone that Darrington would be the next patient. As he left the room, the family all held hands and encircled Darrington as he lay in the hospital bed. After the prayers had gone up, each one gave him a hug and told him that everything would be all right. The Operating Room Nurse came in to get him and he was immediately taken in for surgery.

A few of the family members went to the cafeteria for coffee in hopes of getting rid of some of their nervous energy, while others insisted that they would remain in the waiting room, no matter how long the procedure took. Of course his mother never moved from her chair, but instead she sat like the Virgin Mary and quietly cried out to God for her only son that fought so desperately for his life. During surgery Darrington's father arrived to offer support, as well. The two casually greeted each other, but there was really no conversation.

After a few hours went by, which seemed like an eternity, the surgeon came out and requested to speak with the family of Darrington Lovelace. Everyone anxiously scurried into the small waiting room to hear the report. The doctor explained that several inches of his colon had been removed as it contained numerous cancerous cells. He also indicated that it was possible that Darrington may also be a good candidate for Chemotherapy as a pre-emptive means of addressing the Cancer.

Lynn was curious about the possibility of a colostomy, but the surgeon assured her that there was no need as the colon had been adequately repaired. Before the surgeon left, he indicated that Darrington was currently in the recovery room, and would soon awaken and be able to visit with the family in about an hour. Everyone breathed a sigh of relief, but there was an unspoken apprehension in the air that the nefarious cancer would return. It certainly wasn't the news that everyone wanted to hear, but it was the next best thing. Lynn knew that Chemotherapy would be a rough process, but if that is what Darrington needed to save his life, then that's what would have to be done. We all had the "it is what it is attitude."

Following the recovery, Darrington said he felt okay, but mostly he was relieved that it was over. He knew that he would remain in the hospital for a few more days and then be discharged from the hospital to mentally prepare himself for Chemotherapy. Prior to the Chemotherapy treatment, Darrington was informed that the current hospital was conducting experimental programs that involved cancer patients. Although Darrington was invited to participate in the program, he declined because he felt uncomfortable with the word "experiment." He verbalized having some reservations about the program as he felt that his condition was grave and he just wanted to know for certain that he would be given the proper medications and not risk being given any kind of placebos. I'm really not sure if the experimental program was explained to him in its entirety.

While under the care of the local Oncologist, it was later determined that the aggressive menacing Cancerous tumors had also begun attacking the liver and lung organs as well.

The new information was very difficult to hear since it had only been a few weeks since the removal of a large section of the colon. Right away, Darrington's heart sank lower than the basement, not to mention everyone else's as well. Deep inside everyone's thoughts were the words "death sentence" but of course nobody dared to say it. Everyone wanted to be strong and hopeful for Darrington. Likewise, he wanted to be strong and hopeful for everyone, and especially himself. In his mind, he was pretty much resolved to the fact that there had to be more aggressive treatment elsewhere that perhaps he should at least look into and or take advantage of.

As he began researching alternative programs that were located within and out of State he was intrigued by the television commercial regarding Cancer Center Treatments of America. The closest center was about a four-hour drive away. He phoned the center and spoke to the Admissions Director who was very pleasant. He seemed very pleased with the information that he received as they spoke highly of their success rates. Darrington shared the information with his mother who was also excited and ready to explore new options and chart new territory. His mother knew that Zion Illinois was at least a four-hour drive from where they lived, but it made no difference to her because it was absolutely imperative that her son receive the best possible care.

Darrington was given an appointment to go over and tour the facility and meet with the Admissions Coordinator, Medical Social Workers, etc. They were given a tour of the facility, insurance issues were addressed, and they were informed of any financial assistance programs that were available to them specifically for low income patients. They were even given free tickets to the nearby zoo, which I thought was certainly a nice way to focus on the lighter and pleasant side. Following that meeting, Darrington was scheduled to meet with the Oncologist to determine the direction of his treatment, specific medication regiments, and diet changes that would take place.

After a series of tests, it was confirmed that the Cancer had definitely mushroomed to the liver and also the lungs, but yet the doctors were hopeful that they could help him beat the odds. The Oncologist explained that there were actually three tumors on the liver that they could remove. As far as the lungs were concerned, they intended to perform a series of Chemotherapy treatments, which would hopefully eradicate those dreadful nefarious cells as well.

This second surgery was scheduled for the purpose of removing more than half of the liver organ. Darrington was informed that even though two thirds of his liver would be removed, he was not to worry because the tissues would eventually regenerate within a matter of time. He was warned that he should be careful of the amount of medications he took because most medications were filtered through the liver for processing. Just as before, all immediate family members traveled to Zion to provide love, support and prayers. His father, Darren also managed to get to the center.

Just before surgery, the family all joined hands, and prayed the prayer of healing and faith. Immediately following the prayer, he was taken to the operating room by the nurse. This time the procedure was even more invasive and lasted more hours than before. After several hours, the doctor came out into the waiting room and talked with family about the surgery. He reported that everything had gone well and that he would be available to speak with the family in about an hour, as he was still in recovery.

Everyone rushed to his side to provide support. Although he was able to speak, he was pretty groggy. Most of the family chose to go back to their hotels in order to give him a chance to rest after such an invasive therapy. Because of employment obligations, some family members stayed for only a day or two before returning home. Even though some had to leave, close contact was kept on Darrington via telephone.

Approximately two weeks later, Chemotherapy treatments were scheduled to begin. Darrington's time was designated on a Thursday morning, which meant that his mother or whomever was going to provide transportation had to leave late Wednesday evening in order for him to be present on Thursday morning at 10:00 a.m. Before he could receive Chemotherapy, he had to meet with the Oncologist to test his blood to be sure that his white blood count was within range. This was also a good time for Darrington and his mother to discuss any concerns that they had with the doctor. Once it was determined that his blood levels were within range, he was given permission to proceed with Chemotherapy which was quite a process.

The Chemotherapy treatments were aggressive as they were aimed at destroying the tumors that had been detected on the lungs and anywhere else the cancer might be lurking. Originally Darrington was scheduled to receive treatments every week. If he became too tired, and or too nauseous he was allowed to skip a few weeks of treatment, but later he was put right back on schedule. In the beginning, the treatment regimen was going along very well, his cancer markers were gradually declining, and everyone was very encouraged. On one occasion he was informed that his numbers had almost completely declined ...yeah! Considering the fact that it seemed he had only been prescribed about fifty different pills to treat the symptoms which covered up more symptoms, to cover up even more symptoms and so on, everyone had great expectations. The fact that Darrington experienced severe pill fatigue was just a phase that he would have to endure to reach his healing.

Unfortunately, no matter how low the numbers were, he always said he had a constant aching pain in the abdomen and the lower back. On a scale of one to ten, he said his pain was most always a seven. By the time he took a week or two off to rest from the very stressful chemotherapy, it was time to put his feet back in the stirrups, jump right back on the angry bucking chemo horse and ride again. The next time around, he was told that his cancer markers had taken an upsurge, which made him feel even more guilty for taking the time to get off the enraged minacious chemo ass in the first place. It really seemed that the cancerous bitch had a mind of her own and was absolutely thrilled with the fact that Darrington just couldn't seem to figure out how to get even one step ahead of her. It felt like a rigged game that he just couldn't win.

Nobody seemed to be able to make any helpful suggestions that made any difference; we were all at our wits end. No matter what we tried or suggested, the hostile cancer refused to respond to anything. Oh how we loathed that bitch! In my mind, I could hear Satan laughing hysterically, uncontrollably, insisting that he wanted Darrington to anathematize his Christian faith. The thought of a horse laughing with the sound of a human being made me sick to my stomach, let alone having two heads. Like Job, no matter how discouraged he became, he never said those words.

As time went on, it seemed that the cancer began to proliferate and devour his body even more. No longer was he on the demonic horse, but somehow that horse quickly ran through a window of transmogrify and was now running at a much faster high speed runaway train, which was being driven by the Conductor, Satan himself. It was certainly a mega megillah and required a ton of prayer, as far as I was concerned.

As I prayed, God revealed to me exactly what was happening. Make no mistake, Darrington was never alone as he was constantly surrounded by a host of angels, who were all under the auspices of my Lord and Savior, Jesus Christ. Unfortunately, Darrington was being stalked and tortured by the most audacious deadly and vindictive force on earth. The Devil saw him as easy prey that he could toss to and fro like a baby. Since Darrington wouldn't denounce his faith the devil stepped up the pace. Darrington was now a passenger on an evil and deadly runaway train. I imagined the color of the train as a distinctive dull dreary black with black shades pulled down so that it was literally impossible for anyone to see in or out. I vaguely saw what appeared to be a giant wave of sparks that enveloped the entire train. It was moving so fast that I could barely see the driver, but I was able to determine that it was Satan indeed. His head resembled that of a deadly venomous Cobra snake and all I could see was its slithering tongue moving rapidly in and out, but it was wrapped around something white. *Oh dear Lord! I think he's smokin a joint*, I thought. The train traveled faster and faster as it picked up speed; it appeared as if it was being carried by a whirlwind.

It took no time at all for me to discern that the devil represents nothing short of the bowels of hell that could only be satisfied by spreading sickness, disease, idolatry, hatred, jealousy, into the atmosphere via viscous vomit and putrid defecation.

Botulism, botulism, and more botulism immediately came to my mind. The evil stalker's goal is to entrap and extirpate everyone because they are ignorant and unaware of his trickery that is so magnificently disguised. I hate to give Satan credit, but he is definitely world-renowned for his death and destruction abilities. In spite of his abilities I refuse to wear the masks of sickness, disease, idolatry, hatred, etc. I will rebuke the devil and call him a liar. I will curse him and tell him to take his damn masks back. Even if my physical health declines, I will stay the course. Yes, life is full of negative drama that seems never ending, but I am determined to stay the course. Even though the world continues to rock and reel and quite presumably will fall off the axis; I am planning to stay the course just as Job did!

Selfishness, jealousy, lack of support, all are just ugly tactics that the devil uses to control us. I've witnessed too many individuals who will say with a smile "I can't help you cause I ain't got no money." If you always say you have no money, then I believe that you truly never will have any money, because God blesses the cheerful giver. Certainly we may not all have significant amounts of money to contribute to our friends and neighbors, but that is no excuse to do nothing at all. Perhaps a ride to a medical appointment, $5 - $10 for lunch or gas, mow grass, or even prepare a meal. I really have a hard time believing that we can never spare $5-$10 especially when we somehow miraculously manage to do everything else we want to do.

There were times that Darrington didn't have energy to prepare himself a meal, much less mow grass. He definitely could have really used some help, or even just to know that a friendly visitor would be coming by. I suggest that we wipe that smile off our faces, stop lying and go ahead and cheerfully contribute what little we have and then let's watch God bless us abundantly so that we would not have room enough to receive it.

> *Dear children, let's not merely say that we love each other; let us show the truth by our actions...*
> **1 John 3:18**

Darrington was always willing to contribute what little he had, especially if he knew someone was in need. He had a very kind and giving spirit about him, even before he was diagnosed with cancer.

If we all performed one act of kindness per day, no person would be ever without anything. Let's not use generic statements, "you're in my thoughts and prayers" and not ever follow up with a kind deed. If you know someone has an illness, don't wait until the funeral to stand up in front of the fully-packed church to say how much you loved them when you never did anything. Anybody can recite brilliant speeches and say the nicest words, but we need to do what we can for each other while we can on this side of heaven. Keep in mind that someday we will all experience being a patient and or be immobile and helpless.

Darrington was like any normal individual, innocently strolling through his journey of life, winding through innocuous woods, while admiring a beautiful forest. Of course the paths of sickness and disease were invisible and all he could see was beautiful floridity which nonchalantly lured him into the devil's web. He only saw the good in people and things. He had no idea that such an alluring forest was actually an invitation to disaster. "All must pay some, but some must pay all" certainly held true in this case. Certainly the great "I AM" is mighty and all powerful, but Satan too wants to flex his muscles just as a reminder to us that no one, and I mean no one, is exempt from the spirit of evil.

For the sake of Darrington's protection, we all formed a permanent imaginary prayer circle of support and protection around him in the precious name of Jesus and by his stripes we are healed, I said out loud. We cared less that our circle was no stronger than the weakest link; we just knew that when Lucifer finally drove that damn train over the cliff, we were all going to be piled on top of him to assure that he wasn't going through any of it alone, even if it meant we would have all been slaughtered sheep, that was just how much we loved him.

This vicious violent emotional roller coaster had gone on for nearly three years. The Oncologists worked frantically and desperately tried several methods to halt the High Speed train, but their efforts were doomed. The treatment regiments were constantly mixed and matched in hopes of finding the silver bullet to stop the damn horse. It was somewhat like the matching game, where the cards were overturned until a match was discovered. His life was reduced to somewhat of a matching game.

By this time, Darrington's physical appearance was that of emotional, physical, and mental drain. Once in a great while, he would say he was tired, and or in pain, but not often. If a picture is worth a thousand words, the exhausted look of his eyes clearly showed that his life was literally and slowly being sucked out of him. The once, tall, Hershey dark chocolate, strapping young man, had been reduced to a very weak, frail, depressed, anxious and emotionally broken individual that was barely able to walk. He even owned a wheelchair, which the professionals referred to as the top of the line "Cadillac" walker because it just happened to have a fancy little seat and a basket to carry small items and a set of brakes on the handle bars just in case he was going too fast. Yippee ki-yay!

Over time, the effects of the Chemotherapy in addition to the fact that the cancer was spreading, naturally increased his level of depression and anxiety. He knew that once he received the treatments, the side effects would make him deathly ill, which more often than not landed him in the hospital for two weeks just to stabilize the effects of the Chemo. He once mentioned to me that he needed to see a Psychiatrist to get medication for depression and anxiety in anticipation of the side effects of the Chemotherapy. Very few times did he express the need to take respite breaks from the Chemotherapy because he desperately hoped that his numbers would begin to decline.

Regardless of how sick he felt, he always tried to be positive while praying for a miracle. If the thought of death entered his mind, he and the family quickly put it out by reciting biblical scriptures, or singing spiritual songs, etc. Out of sight, out of mind was how he and the family coped with his Cancer; besides, he was much too young to die. To entertain the idea was simply too much for him or anyone in the family to deal with. Quite frankly, nobody wanted to let go, especially without giving it every ounce of effort that we had. Darrington was too young and besides that, we, meaning the family considered ourselves as Christian soldiers fighting in God's army.

Darrington usually left for Chicago on Wednesday afternoon. Following the treatments, it was usually late Thursday evening before all the intravenous fluids finished. By that time, Lynn had sat and spent quality time with Darrington, followed by meetings with doctors, socials workers and neither she nor Darrington was in any shape to make the four-hour drive back to Michigan. Most often, they headed back home on Friday morning. This meant they always wound up smack dab in the middle of all the treacherous Chicago traffic, which included a lot of repetitive stopping, starting, slowing down. It really did a number on the brakes of her automobile. Sometimes he was so sick to his stomach that the driver would have to stop the car to let him vomit. The cost of the trips turned out to be very high because of the tolls, round trip gas prices, hotels, meals, wear and tear on the car, etc. It was certainly a very overwhelming ordeal.

In the beginning, the Cancer Center Treatments of American provided adequate financial assistance, but understandably it wasn't ongoing as they were obligated to help as many patients as they could. Although Darrington's income was minuscule he did the best he could to pay for the trips and so did his mother who eventually had to resort to use Family Medical Leave benefits where she received no income at all. Initially she was able to withstand the time away from her job and all of the expenses, but as time went on, her financial ship sank as well. Family members helped out as much as possible, but it eventually took a toll on everyone who would somehow continue to do whatever they could for him.

CHAPTER EIGHT

HE DANCED HIS ASS OFF

During the summer of the third year of illness, there was a Family Reunion held in Florida, which Darrington indicated that he really wanted to attend as he knew there would be relatives that he had never been formally introduced to. Although nobody verbalized the words, obviously everyone had the feeling that it may be Darrington's last opportunity to attend a reunion, especially on this side of heaven. I wasn't able to attend due to my work schedule; but I was ecstatic that he and his mother and sisters were planning to go and made arrangements for him, as well. No one really spoke much of the reunion when they returned, other than to say that they all had a good time.

Fortunately, I ran into Nellie, an elderly cousin, who also attended the reunion. Nellie had the biggest grin on her face and she wasted no time telling me that Darrington won a really nice flat screen television and most of all, she said, "I watched that boy dance his ass off." It was no surprise that she found the whole experience to be pretty remarkable and such an enjoyable performance. I chuckled; but I was thankful that he was able to make the trip and thoroughly enjoy himself as well. I later asked him about it, and he said, "Auntie Gladys, I don't know what happened; I just felt like my cancer was gone." It was short-lived, but at least God gave him a chance to enjoy something special. "You too deserve to have something in this world," I said.

Summer was nearly over and Darrington had recently

returned from an absolutely fabulous Family Reunion in Florida. It seemed that within 24-48 hours that crazy cancerous bitch brought her ass right on back too. By this time, Darrington was heading into his fourth year, and he said his pain level was no better; as a matter of fact, it was worse. Somewhere in the chaotic process he decided to obtain a Marijuana card that would allow him to legally use at his discretion. I'm not sure exactly how much relief he actually received, because he never really seemed comfortable. I think it was one of those simple pleasures he found along his journey that he thought would bring comfort.

Darrington could most always be found lying either on the living room couch or in bed all bundled up like a baby. He often complained of being cold, even if everyone else was hot. By this time, he didn't have much strength or the desire to prepare himself a meal. He relied upon his family members for assistance. Sometimes he would spend a few days with his younger sister, but there were also times when he was left alone because everyone had to work.

If I knew he was alone at his mother's house, I would make it a point to go and sit with him at least for a few hours to keep him company and or to buy him lunch from Subway restaurant, which he really loved. Turkey sandwiches were his favorite. Regardless of how rotten he felt, he always perked up a bit when he had company, especially if there was a nice little snack involved. Occasionally, when he could muster up enough strength, he chose to ride along to go to the restaurant to purchase his own sandwich. No matter how rotten he felt and or how little money he had, he insisted on buying me a sandwich or strawberry licorice too. He knew I loved licorice more than a sub.

Unfortunately, the Oncologists were never able to bring his pain under control, which harrowed him terribly. He was forced to wear a pain pump that contained Dalaudin, which seemed to be the only medication that kept the pain at bay. My daughter, Monique who had also received Dalaudin in the past, described it as the "big gun." Many years ago, she developed Crohn's disease and Dalaudin was one of the few medications that seemed to control her pain as well.

Nevertheless, the doctors were very uncomfortable about leaving Darrington on such high lethal dosages for long periods as they felt either his heart would stop and or he would just stop breathing. Eventually there was discussion about the possibility of Darrington having a surgically implanted pump that he could control independently. Of course by this time, the doctors were hinting that perhaps he should also consider Hospice. Regardless of how bad the situation seemed, Darrington refused to consider Hospice as he believed in God for a complete recovery. He was really saddened and taken aback by the fact that the doctors were practically at the end of their treatment options. On several occasions he said, "I just don't want everybody to give up on me."

Even though the doctors tried to present Hospice as another form of treatment, Darrington wasn't buying into it, neither was his mother who was also in somewhat of a stage of denial. She wasn't going to insist that Darrington man up and be realistic because she knew he was her only son and a competent adult who just happened to be watching his life slip away like sand flowing through an hourglass. For Christ sake, it was her only son, how could she just sit back and let nature take its course without trying to pull out all the stops.

For God so loved the world that he gave his only begotten son, meant nothing to her at the time, it was simply a good scripture in the Bible, John 3:16. By now his body began to slowly retain fluid, his face began to look really plump.

Because the Oncologists felt they had exhausted all regiments of treatments, they later took more of an aggressive stance; but, they also tried to be compassionate, while saying that no further treatments would be performed at the center. And any other comfort measures should be sought at a facility closer to home. Although Darrington knew they were right, he just wasn't ready to accept the fact that he was running out of options. It was just too big of a lump to push down his throat. He continued to grasp at straws while trying to cope with the never-ending depressing news. What you gonna do now? Them damn doctors done threw yo ass under the bus, Satan whispered in Darrington's ear. He was too nice of a guy to ever say the words, but it's exactly how he felt inside as he mentally licked his wounds and crawled away. Meanwhile, his pride was rapidly vanishing.

I'm sure Darrington felt as though he was a hamster running and running on the exercise wheel, going nowhere fast, and certainly making no progress. The faster he ran, the worse he became, he didn't know what to do to try to help himself, nor did anyone else. Somebody, anybody, help me please, I'm running out of time, he thought.

Because he had reached the end of his treatment at Cancer Center Treatment of America, he was at least given the option of having an electronic pain pump surgically implanted. The only problem was that when the portable pain pump was discontinued, and the electronic pump was implanted, the current high dosages of medication didn't automatically transfer over, but instead had to be reset to begin from the lowest dosage and work upward in small increments. He was told that he would need to make weekly trips back to Chicago to have the dosages slowly increased.

After the surgery he had quite an ugly scar that began at the middle of his back and went around to the middle of his stomach. In addition, he had a hand held device that he was instructed to hold up to his abdomen before pressing a button in order to receive a small dosage of medication, which he said felt as though he got no relief at all. Of course he had pain medication that he could also take by mouth, but those could only be taken every four to six hours. Unfortunately, his options were limited. He actually did make a few trips back to the Center to have the dosages increased, but clearly it wasn't enough to soothe and quiet the raging angry pain. I wondered if perhaps the whole surgical process wasn't a ploy to nudge him into receiving Hospice services.

Because neither Darrington nor his mother was ready to accept Hospice Services, she made contact with a local doctor whom she had known for quite some time. The doctor reluctantly agreed to assume responsibilities for his care, but more, he also saw a very desperate mother who wasn't ready to let go of her son and will him to die. The physician willingly received report from the Illinois Oncologist and was determined to do whatever he could to help his new patient. Though Darrington actually had consultations with the two local physicians, he was not able to receive the particular recommended Chemotherapy because his cancer had metastasized into other organs, nor did he seem very interested at the time as well. At this time, he had received no Chemotherapy in about three almost four months.

Time marched right along and so did his level of organ deterioration. Fluid slowly continued to pool over his body from the top of his head to the sole of his feet. His entire body had drastically increased in size considering his normal weight. Fortunately, the doctors were smart enough to input a catheter which allowed him to urinate, otherwise the swelling would have closed off and stopped his ability to pass urine. For some reason his left side seemed to have a bit more fluid than the right. He had a very difficult time ambulating, not to mention the fact that he was extremely uncomfortable and still experiencing quite a bit of pain.

The last time he came home from the Cancer Center, he had some difficulty getting out of the car. As usual, he was exhausted from such a long ride home, not to mention his medical condition. He was so drained that he sat in the car for a short while to gather his thoughts before coming inside. He required a bit of assistance to get into the house and up the stairs in order to get into his bed. Because of the vast amount of fluid retention, it was very difficult to bend his legs. As he tried to climb the stairs, he nearly fell twice. By this time, he was in tears, but he kept going. When he finally got to the top of the stairs and sat down on the bed, I put my arms around him and just held him while he sobbed. As he laid on his bed he asked if he could be propped up with pillows so he could be a bit more comfortable. He mentioned that he was having quite a bit of pain in his lower back as well. The television was turned on to his favorite shows and he calmed down and tried to focus on something other than how rotten he felt.

CHAPTER NINE

TURTLE DOVE HOLISTIC CARE

Darrington asked me if I would contact a very familiar friend, Karla Anderson, Registered Nurse, as he knew she was the Director of the local Turtle Dove Holistic and Wellness Center. Darrington knew that Karla would focus not only on the Cancer, but instead on the whole body and work to bring the body back to balance, which she knew was a process and would require time. From a holistic point of view, once all of the deficiencies have been addressed and under control, then the illnesses will go away on their own because there would be nothing to disguise them. She was well aware that Darrington's condition was grave and it would be nothing short of an uphill battle; but she was determined to give it her best effort. He accepted the fact that he would receive no further treatment at the CCTA as "he had failed" all available treatments based on their standards. Although it made no difference, I just wished they would have reworded the statement differently by saying, the "treatments failed Darrington."

Karla was more than happy to see Darrington, even on weekends, evenings, etc. Seeing Karla was like a breath of fresh air, a burst of energy that he needed. Karla was well aware that he needed extremely exigent care as he was in dire straits. She had a combination of treatments that she was very eager to try in order to start the process of bringing his whole body back into balance. For once, Darrington had hope. Instead of being told that there were no more available treatments for him to fail, he was now off the deadly beaten path heading right into that fabulous busy intersection of hope! He followed Karla's advice and actually began feeling a bit better mentally and physically. Not only were his spirits were lifted, he was actually beginning to lose a bit of the fluid which was due to a few Foot Soak treatments. After about two weeks of receiving treatment from the Holistic Center it seemed that things just might be starting to move in the right direction.

Late one evening Darrington began feeling very uncomfortable. He indicated that his pain seemed to be increasing and he seemed to be having some difficulty breathing. His body temperature was rapidly changing from hot to cold. One minute he wanted a blanket the next minute he wanted the fan on high. I saw the look of worry and extreme desperation on his face that will forever remain etched in my mind. We all knew that something was definitely wrong. His mother put her arms around him and hugged him as she tried to bring comfort, but she too had the same look of fear upon her face as well. This process went on for about an hour which seemed like an eternity. All the while he was constantly trying to get some relief from his implanted pain pump that he said seemed completely worthless as he constantly pressed the button. He continued as long as he could but finally said he couldn't stand the pain any longer. Frantically, he cried out in pain as he begged to go to the hospital. As the pain intensified, so did the magnitude of his cries. His mother tried to console him by massaging his back and increasing some of his supplements, but nothing helped.

Finally, a phone call was made for the Ambulance to come immediately without the sirens or the lights. His mother had to swallow very hard because she knew exactly what was happening and what the next step would be. She felt as though she was on a cliff, barely hanging on to her son who was slowly slipping away from her grip regardless of her prayers or her efforts. It seemed that the tighter she held on, the more he slipped away. The Ambulance finally arrived and prepared him for the ride to the hospital. Because his body had retained so much fluid, it was very difficult for him to walk down the stairs to the ambulance. The stairs made it impossible to use the stretcher. Finally, he was assisted into the ambulance which was terribly painful for him. After he was made comfortable they attempted to start an Intravenous drip; but because his veins were in such bad shape from years of pokes and prods, it was nearly impossible to find a decent one. It was somewhat like looking for a needle in a haystack.

Lynn was furious as she knew Darrington was extremely uncomfortable, and needed to receive immediate treatment for pain and comfort. She mentioned that she could have put him in her car and had him at the hospital by now. She tried to be calm and not insult the Emergency Medical Staff; but she had to bite her tongue as she really felt they were incompetent. In their defense, they did mention that they were short staffed and were required to cover a broader area. Because she had worked many years as a Phlebotomist and a Nurse, she felt that she could have found a vein in no time at all. After about thirty minutes, they finally pulled off and she followed behind them in her car. With the worst thoughts running through her mind, she tried to remain positive, but also knew that Darrington was actually one step closer to the grave.

Leo Sullivan

I was suddenly reminded of a former friend, Leo Sullivan, who is now deceased. Leo was diagnosed with severe Diverticulitis which occurred as a result of him being a prisoner of war for many months as a young man. He mentioned that the living conditions were extremely perilous as he was forced to live on a starvation diet, which nearly caused his demise. With God's help he lived through it. Leo was a great friend and I frequented his apartment as often as I had the chance. Other than his warm and friendly demeanor, I recall that he was often very uncomfortable and unable to control his bowels. Though he was retired at that time, he said the only way he had previously been able to work and make a living for himself and his wife, Mary, was to take Paregoric which the doctor regularly prescribed for him; otherwise he would have been totally disabled.

Once Leo retired, and his doctor passed away, he was on his own to make the best of his life and to try to enjoy his family. There were times when I would visit Leo and he would spend practically the entire visit in the bathroom. Though he apologized profusely; he just couldn't control his bowels. Even though Leo spent half his life experiencing nothing but pain and discomfort he was determined to enjoy life as best he could. Darrington reminded me of him in some way. He too was determined to have some sort of enjoyment in his life. Leo had a great sense of humor but he never failed to say, "Gladys, I got one foot in the grave and the other foot on a banana peel." We both laughed but knew his condition was severe as well.

From Hospital to Hospice House

The next day we went to the hospital to visit Darrington who seemed to be resting comfortably in bed. His appearance was fair, but at least all the fluid that he previously carried had been drained by the doctor during a procedure to make him more comfortable. Lynn was told that a total of ten pounds of fluid had been removed from his body. He currently received oxygen and what seemed like several bags of intravenous hydration and pain medication for comfort. Darrington was very fatigued and resolved to the fact that the current doctors strongly suggested that he be admitted to the local Hospice House. Both he and his mother reluctantly agreed to follow their recommendations.

Darrington could see that his condition had declined beyond his mother's ability to care for him at home. He knew that his pain was too great, nor was he physically able to make any more trips to Chicago to have his surgically implanted pump adjusted. His spirit was severely damaged nor did he seem to have any more fight inside. Though he was damaged he had not totally lost the will to live, because he refused to sign DNR (do not resuscitate) orders. Physically, mentally and emotionally, he still felt that he had a very slight chance. He knew that there were sometimes Hospice graduates and could have easily been one. If his faith could have been measured, surely it would have been at least as big as a mustard seed.

The Hospice Director urged Lynn to overrule his wishes, but she refused as she felt that he was competent and able to make informed decisions. Darrington's preference was not to be sedated beyond his ability to speak and be aware of his surroundings. He wanted to be able to greet his family and friends that came to see him. As a result, there was just a bit of friction between how he wanted his pain managed and what the Hospice staff were accustomed to providing the patients. Nevertheless, they were able to meet Darrington's needs. Although he never signed DNR orders, he was made as comfortable as he wanted to be. Originally Lynn was informed that Darrington had only a matter of weeks to live, based on his CAT (computerized axial tomography) scan. A day or two later, she was informed that the Cancer cells had mushroomed into the neck area and he had only a few days to live. Of course the news hit her like a ton of bricks. How could she tell her son that he would be dead within a few days, but then again, how could she not?

Darrington knew he was at the Hospice House because his condition had declined, but yet he felt as though he still had a chance. A visitor that he knew came in to say hello and asked if he had been talking to God? Yes, he responded. She asked him what advice God had given him about his condition. He said, "God told me not to worry about it." He still believed that God had the last say and would heal him regardless of what the doctors at the facility said, who he respected and graciously thanked for their care.

Consequently, Lynn decided not to tell him as it would serve no purpose for him to know that he was even closer to death than they had imagined. She too believed that God could turn any situation around if he chose to do so, but why wasn't he choosing to do it for him, for her, for the family? My faith wasn't perfect, but I know for sure that I had the faith of a mustard seed, I thought.

During his Hospice stay, he received a visit from two staff

members from Oaklawn Homecare, Shelly and Lori who had developed a good relationship with him; and he really appreciated them and their services as well. During their visit, they mentioned that they looked forward to seeing him on the other side. He didn't really have any comments until they left, but he asked me if I thought he was dying. I told him that anything was possible as his life was still in God's hands. He was very content and said "I don't know what they're talkin bout cause I aint gonna die."

All family members were informed as to the amount of time the doctors had given him and all were told not to disclose the information. I do recall on one occasion when Darrington was having lunch and he looked directly at me and said, "It's okay that I'm here because I need a lot of help." It was almost as if he wanted me to approve and or confirm his thoughts. I was hesitant to respond because his mother had instructed us all not to provide him with specific information about his length of time left here on earth. As I look back, I really don't recall saying too much, but instead, I just gave him a warm gentle smile.

Even though Darrington only had a couple of days to live, his appetite seemed fair, he was alert, oriented, and able to make decisions independently and talk with family. He had a very difficult time ambulating because by this time, he appeared to be carrying even more fluid than was previously drained while he was in the hospital. When he ambled, he had somewhat of a penguin's Gait. As if that wasn't bad enough he had about ten feet of oxygen tubing which was easily entangled. Lynn remained with him as much as she could, but there were times that she needed to run some errands.

CHAPTER TEN

HOSPICE HOUSE

One day Lynn asked me if I could stay with him while she ran some errands. I happily agreed as I had not had a chance to be alone with Darrington since he arrived at the Hospice Home. Towards the beginning of the visit, he seemed okay. His pain wasn't too bad. The nurses came in every twenty minutes or sooner to determine if he needed anything. He was as comfortable as possible, he said. Without actually verbalizing the fact that he knew he wasn't going to live much longer, he asked me if I would write a book about his life. He stressed the fact that he just didn't want to be forgotten. He and I embraced for what seemed like an eternity. Of course I'll write a book about your life and I plan to start a Scholarship Memorial for you as well, I said. He seemed very pleased and began to provide specific information and pictures that he wanted included. I promised him that he needn't worry about anything as it would be my pleasure to bring both the book and the Scholarship Memorial to fruition. He seemed relieved as he knew that his wishes would be brought to fruition. Neither of us ever said the word "death," by that time it seemed to be a mutual understanding.

Shortly following the conversation, Darrington leaned back in attempt to take a short nap. He was never able to fall asleep as he said he felt a bit more painful and uncomfortable than usual. He called for the nurse who immediately came and gave him a small dosage of medication. Since he didn't want to be heavily sedated, he received the minimal dosages of medications. He tried to get comfortable in bed by fluffing his pillows and fixing the sheets, but said he felt minimal relief which only seemed to last a few seconds. He rang for the nurse again, who immediately came and gave him just a bit more.

The process quickly started over again, except after about three minutes, he let out a very gut wrenching scream from the top of his lungs as a result of pain which he said was now worse than ever before. He began to moan, cry and sweat profusely. The nurse came running in and gave him more medication. It seemed that he just couldn't get comfortable and continued to scream out in pain, which made me very uncomfortable. The degree at which he screamed sounded as if he was being brutally murdered and literally amputated limb by limb. By this time, the nurse remained by his side, giving an even higher dosage of pain medication as needed. The nurse's forbearance in caring for Darrington was commendable. She explained that the medication had to be dispersed slowly so that his heart wouldn't immediately stop. Because Lynn had left instructions for his sheets to be changed, the nurse asked if I could help him stand while she changed the sheets. It only took about two minutes, but it was obvious that Darrington experienced such severe excruciating pain and when he stood it seemed to be ten times worse, based on the level of his screams.

He was put back to bed immediately after the clean sheets were on. *Why the hell didn't they just roll him in bed instead of having him stand up?* I thought. Because he was in so much pain, it probably would have made no difference anyway. It seemed as though he was about to pass out from being in so much pain, which continued to increase and yet would react to the medication for only a few minutes. He only received brief moments of relief with each injection.

As his eyes rolled back and forth, he somehow managed to look into my eyes and ask, "How is everything going"? "I am okay but right now you're more important," I said. Even during the midst of his dying process, he still worried more about others than himself. *What a saint*, I said to myself. I could tell that he was becoming very lethargic, and exhausted from the pain, which had taken a toll on his fragile body. He woke up for a second and cried out "Thank you Jesus."

Shortly thereafter, he cried out for his earthly father who was not present. "Hey dad," he yelled. I knew he was either confused and or dreaming because his father had not yet been to the Hospice House to visit with him since he had been there. If there was ever a time for his dad to be around, it was then, but he wasn't. Once again, he wasn't there when Darrington really needed him. However, he did manage to come up and visit towards the very end of his life. Because he no longer drove, he had to have friends transport him wherever he went. Darrington's body was now a limp noodle that was sprawled across the bed. I had to struggle to hold back the tears, not to mention that fact that my nerves were completely shot. All of a sudden I felt an adrenaline surge. I became terribly anxious and sweaty about the level of pain that Darrington currently experienced. I tried to massage his back and the soles of his feet with Essential oils as I consoled him but nothing helped. I just wanted the pain to STOP. In my mind I kept repeating the words "he's suffering too much, we don't let animals suffer like this."

A weird feeling came over me. My body tingled from top to bottom as a result of being in such a stressful situation. Fortunately, I wasn't a smoker because I'm sure I would have smoked a whole pack of cigarettes and or taken a handful of Xanex to calm my nerves. *How could any human being endure that level of pain*, I thought? Finally, after about forty minutes, it seemed that Darrington had received enough medication to quiet the pain at least for a while. He slept and I breathed a sigh of relief. I too sat back in the chair as I felt like an ocean of stress had just left my body.

Although he was quiet, the sound of his screams will forever remain etched in my mind. The two childbirths that I had in no way compared to the level of pain that I just watched Darrington endure. As it turned out I realized that I was nothing more than a wimp; I didn't even want to be awake for any part of the birthing process for either of my children. I recalled the conversation that I had with the Obstetrician from my first pregnancy. He was a young doctor, very intelligent and he proceeded to tell me that I looked like a strong enough person to deliver the child naturally.

That was all I needed to hear, I kindly thanked him for his service, walked out the door and immediately phoned an alternative obstetrician who would agree to give me as much pain medication as I needed. I never even called the guy back to explain my issues or even to cancel my next appointment as I had no use for him. If I could have talked the doctors into putting me to sleep while the babies were born, that would have been just fine with me because I didn't want to feel even an ounce of pain or discomfort, regardless of how the medication would have affected the unborn children. I was only concerned with my pain tolerance, which was lower than the basement; and the unborn babies would just have to manage on their own until I birthed them. Needless to say, neither of my doctors would hear of it.

For a few seconds I honestly thought of how Jesus must have felt while being severely beaten all night long and finally nailed to an old rugged cross that he himself had been mandated to carry. All of a sudden a silence came over me and I had no words to say. I thought of all the times I had complained about what or how real my pain felt. Until then, I had never witnessed any human being experience that level of pain! "Knock him out with everything you've got" was what I really wanted to say to the nurses, but; I had too much respect for him to ever cross that line. He was young, but clearly he was able to make informed decisions.

> *Pain and suffering have come into your life, but remember pain, sorrow, suffering are but the kiss of Jesus-a sign that you have come so close to Him that He can kiss you.*
>
> *-Mother Teresa*

The nurse thanked me for my help and quietly left the room for a short while urging me to call her if Darrington needed anything. I couldn't speak for anyone else, but I could certainly attest to the fact that Darrington had definitely been kissed by Jesus and all of his disciples many times over, especially on that particular afternoon. After about a half hour, I thought I should go home. Lynn had not yet returned, but I was beginning to feel anxious again. Darrington seemed to be resting quietly, and I knew that he was in good hands.

Honestly, I didn't think I could handle another episode like that.

The ride home seemed endless. I rolled the window down to get some fresh air as I needed to feel the wind on my face. I inhaled and exhaled several times taking deep appreciative breaths. I could feel the tightness roaming about my neck and shoulders. As the wind gently massaged my face, I felt my eyes fill with tears and slowly stream down my face. By this time, my vision began to blur and I could barely see the other drivers. *You better stop crying before you have a serious accident and then you'll be laid up in the hospital*, I thought to myself. I quickly but gently wiped the tears away and turned the radio on to my favorite Sirius XM Christian radio station. I felt that I could definitely use a little spiritual uplifting. I drove and drove, but I just couldn't seem to get home fast enough. I just wanted to blink my eyes and magically arrive home. Finally, I arrived home and entered the house, ran straight into my bedroom and collapsed into the bed as I tried to digest what I had just witnessed. I couldn't think, nor did I have the energy to pray. I desperately needed the holy spirit to intercede for me. I fell asleep out of sheer exhaustion.

The next day I called Lynn to find out how he was feeling. Lynn said he wasn't feeling too bad. Darrington had a good breakfast and a decent lunch. He was able to sit up and talk with his siblings, as well. That's good, I responded. I won't come today, I'll visit tomorrow, and I'll bring Jim with me, I said. I didn't dare tell her that my nerves were still very much on edge as a result of the day before. As long as he wasn't alone, that was good enough for me.

CHAPTER ELEVEN

SILENCED FOREVER

The next morning, I went to work, as usual. I forgot that I previously committed to help out at the National Alliance Mental Illness fundraiser. On the way home I received a phone call from his sister, Jaquita. Darrington's heart stopped and he's on his way to the hospital, she said. I'm on my way too, I responded. It was at least a forty-minute ride, which seemed to take forever. *Poor Darrington, why didn't they just let him go*, I thought. *Even if they resuscitate him, the quality of his life is poor, nor is there anything positive for him to look forward to*, I thought.

Regardless, Lynn was determined to respect the wishes of her son, in spite of her own feelings which I totally respected. Consequently, Darrington was transported to the hospital and resuscitated, as he requested. Although the medical staff worked diligently resuscitating him several times, apparently he just couldn't hold on. The mighty risen Savior said, "no more."

> *God's finger touched him, and he slept.*
> — **Alfred Lord Tennyson**

> *See now that I myself am He! There is no God besides me. I put to death and I bring to life, I have wounded and I will heal, and no one can deliver out of my hand.*
> — **Deuteronomy 32:39**

The drive to the hospital took about forty minutes indeed, plus another ten minutes to stop for gas. When I finally reached the hospital, Darrington's oldest sister, Jaquita was sitting quietly outside the room holding her small child. As I approached her, she stared sadly into my eyes and said, "He is gone." Tears streamed down her face. "Oh dear God," I responded. I proceeded into the room to view the body. Sitting up against the wall, I saw Lynn and her youngest daughter Bari, both in tears and totally exhausted, as if the wind had been knocked out of their sails. Darrington's body lay lifeless on the table. His eyes were closed, and blood continued to slowly trickle from both nostrils. Lynn constantly wiped the blood away and placed socks on his feet as if to keep him warm. Even though he lay dead, the motherly instincts continued and become even stronger.

As I briefly visually scanned his body, I noticed that there was not one section that had been untouched from the cancer and its evil side effects. His arms were terribly bruised from top to bottom, and veins had obviously collapsed from years of pokes and prods from the needles. His flesh bore the scars of many surgical procedures that were performed in attempt to decrease pain and eradicate the cancer. The port, which was previously used for Chemotherapy bulged from his chest, and several pounds of fluid distributed itself all over his body; but the right side was noticeably more swollen than the left.

At least it's all over, I thought. In my mind and in my heart I cried uncontrollably. I wanted to cry but for some strange reason, I just couldn't push anything out. I kissed his forehead several times and told him that I loved him and that I was so sorry. I was simultaneously crushed, but yet ecstatic for

Darrington. As much as my heart ached, I was relieved that his discomfort, his ceaseless pain, endless pills, boundless needle pokes and prods, infinite doctor appointments, restless sleepless nights, vomiting, headaches, monotonous trips over the highways, was ALL OVER!

Though we were all absolutely exhausted, we felt like we failed him. One minute he was present and the next minute he was a memory. The hourglass was completely empty and he was forever silenced. Never again, would we hear his laugh or see his smile or enjoy his silly sense of humor. Darrington had been seized, slowly enervated and finally eviscerated by the awful cancer. It seemed so unreal, almost as if we were in a bad dream and were waiting for someone to wake us. *Oh dear God, let this be a dream*, I thought, but it wasn't. No one knew quite what to say.

Occasionally, the nurses would come in to ask if anyone needed anything. The Hospital Chaplin came in to offer counseling and prayer, as well as the Pastor from Darrington's own church. His father, Darren and also many other family members who were able to get to the hospital. Lynn and her daughters graciously thanked the staff for their efforts. Many staff members expressed condolences and hugged the family, as they were coworkers of Lynn and they seemed to greatly sympathize with the family.

After the crowd thinned a bit, I sat down with the family and waited for the mortician, I could clearly feel Darrington's presence in the room. There was a very surreal feeling in the atmosphere. With all my heart, I believe that his spirit aroused and he too was able to observe his physical body and the appalling magnitude of damage caused by the evil and cancerous demon. I could strongly sense that God had honored him and given him a choice to either continue living on earth, or to become totally spiritually free.

Though he was physically deceased; he was spiritually aware of his surroundings. Imaginably he hugged each of us and told us not to be sad because he was no longer in pain. Perchance he tried to tell us that this world was never his home; but now he would go to his new home and live in that glorious mansion in the sky. It was at that point that I realized why I had not been able to cry; his warm and gentle spirit was present and I had a strong gut feeling that he felt great! Indeed, Darrington had walked among us that day and it was very comforting; there was no reason to cry.

It had been at least a three hour wait before the mortician finally arrived. He was very apologetic as he explained that he was on another call, but assured Lynn that he would take very good care of her son. He also indicated that he would contact her in the morning for the purpose of making the funeral arrangements. As the staff and the mortician prepared the body for travel, the first step included placing Darrington inside a white plastic body bag which was snuggly zipped, followed by placing him inside another heavier dark blue body bag which was also zipped closed. Last, the body was then covered by a heavy but soft plushy purple cloth as if to disguise the body which was most likely to deter any suspicions that may have occurred from other patients or their families.

The mortician quickly and quietly rolled the stretcher out of the hospital.

As the mortician rolled the body out, the family members sobbed even more as they knew it was just another step closer towards the end. Even though Darrington was dead, we could still physically touch his body. Seeing him rolled away seemed so final and of course we were in no way ready for closure.

It was clearly after midnight; the mortician had just left the hospital with the body. Lynn wanted to return to the Hospice House to gather all of Darrington's belongings. I offered to drive because I knew she was in no shape to be driving around at that time. When we arrived, Lynn sobbed and was immediately drawn to lay on the bed where Darrington had spent the last week of his life, in attempt to be close to him once more. Obviously she was extremely grief-stricken and unable to focus.

I continued to gather the belongings and carry them out to the car while some of the members of the staff casually came in to express condolences. They had all spent quality time with him. One nurse made the comment that Darrington was now free to dance all over heaven. Lynn seemed to really appreciate all the warm hugs and genuine concern. The drive home was completely silent. What was there to say? Darrington was dead and no longer in the land of the living. The only thing that came to mind was the scripture:

> ***I have fought the good fight, I have finished the race, I have kept the faith.***
>
> **- 2 Timothy 4:7**

Surely Darrington had given it all he had and so did we, I thought to myself. By the time we arrived home, the sun was just coming up and I could hear the birds singing. *At least the birds have a reason to sing,* I thought. I would have loved to know what they could have possibly been singing about at that time; but then again, perhaps it was God's way of telling us that heaven was rejoicing over a new angel that had come home. We proceeded to take most of Darrington's belongings out of the car before we went to bed out of sheer exhaustion.

The next day would prove to be a continuation of even more stress. There were funeral arrangements to be made, phone calls to make, family members to notify. It seemed that the pendulum swung from one extreme to the other. In the midst of grieving, Lynn and her daughters did their best to plan the church service they felt would best represent Darrington. Needless to say they were exceedingly overwhelmed and fatigued; nevertheless, they were determined to get through such a harrowing ordeal. Because Darrington had gained so much weight as a result of all the fluid retention he needed a larger suit. Lynn needed to go shopping for that, as well as shop for Mama who was now diagnosed with Alzheimer and required constant supervision.

The fact that Mama's Alzheimer was at such an advanced state, was actually somewhat bittersweet. As it turned out, she wasn't unable to comprehend that her only grandson that she helped raise had passed away. It seemed that the only thing that stood out in her mind was that there was definitely going to be a church service and she was adamant that she would need to have her Bible in hand. Even in the face of Alzheimer, that particular attribute had not changed.

Whenever she went to church she wouldn't hear of going without her Bible and a few soft tissues to stuff in her purse.

The funeral was very nicely arranged. Somehow Lynn and the girls managed to pull it off without a hitch. I thought the mortician did a wonderful job with Darrington's appearance considering that the cancer had done quite a number on him; he was just as handsome as ever. I could never understand why he had never lost his hair. I recall times that he felt completely rotten, but yet he somehow managed to get himself to the local barber to get his hair cut. Nevertheless, the long four-year battle with the barbarous cancer wreaked havoc on his body; but not once did he ever complain or experience hair loss, which always looked fantastic regardless of how sick he felt. Perhaps it was one of those simple pleasures that God gives us all, regardless of our situations.

The color of the casket was a pretty medium blue trimmed in silver. His attire complemented the casket very well. He wore a beautiful blue tweed suit jacket and dark blue slacks. His shirt underneath was light blue which really enhanced the jacket. I wanted him to wear something of mine, so I contributed a small gold cross with a tiny diamond in the middle. His hair was precisely trimmed just as he always wore it. He truly looked as if he was just taking a nice long nap. The immediate family members were all dressed in various shades of blue that displayed their support to Darrington even in his death. The casket was surrounded by several bouquets of fresh cut roses, daisies, carnations, and a few live plants as well.

The local Grace Temple Church of God in Christ was practically filled to capacity with many people that knew Darrington as a child and had the opportunity to watch him grow up to be a fine young man. It felt as if the entire community of Albion came out to provide support and offer condolences, as well as several family members who traveled from out of State. The two vocalists were awesome and the Pastor even sang a short segment from a familiar song as well as performed a very heartfelt eulogy. Darrington would have absolutely loved such an outpour of support and concern that was shown to his family.

Following the funeral, the body was carefully loaded into a beautiful white Hearse by the Pall Bearers before proceeding to Albion Memory Gardens cemetery where he would be laid to rest. The graveside service took place inside the cemetery Chapel which was short and sweet; the environment seemed very surreal. By the end of the service heavy raindrops began to fall. Very few people had umbrellas, but most didn't, nor did they seemed to care. It was rather disappointing because it discouraged the bereaved from spending ample time in the cemetery. Clearly the temperature dropped at least ten degrees. Even though the temperature seemed to drastically drop, the rain showed no signs of letting up.

The family stood and watched as the casket was very meticulously lowered into the ground. With each three inch drop, the gravediggers paused to assess and assure that the casket specifically lined up with the liner of the vault. Once in place, the lid of the vault could be clearly seen which was beautiful, as Darrington's name was on a silver plate which was engraved in gold. By this time practically everyone had gone except the immediate family. As the rain continued, the wind blew even harder.

As I stood waiting for the body to be lowered into the ground, my mind wandered and I thought of one of my past trips to the island of Jamaica which is a rainy climate. Although Jamaica is a rather poor country, the natives are very kind. The Jamaicans had no issue with the rain and as a matter a fact they seemed to love it, Ya Mon! "Liquid sunshine" is the term used for rain. As my attention was redirected to the funeral, I suddenly felt better about the rain and less concerned about the cold. Nevertheless, Lynn and the two girls huddled closely under an umbrella while dropping yellow roses onto the top of the vault.

The cold literally had no impact upon us as we stood over the body for several minutes longer before slowly walking away. It was extremely difficult to and walk away from the casket because even though he was no longer alive; we knew that the next time we visited the cemetery the only thing they would see was a five-foot dirt covered area where he lay six feet underneath. The fact that we would see him again in heaven was really a rather minuscule thought at the time.

The Repast was held at the local Charles Snyder Community building and was very nice as well. The people in the community came together and really worked hard to donate food, drinks and desserts. The dinner consisted of a light chicken luncheon. There were all kinds of family pictures on the wall for everyone to enjoy and reminisce. Darrington's cousin, Shafton Dunklin had previously compiled quite a few family pictures and dance performances, into a very nice musical video. It was awesome. Just watching all the dance performances brought back many memories. As usual, when he started dancing, everyone stopped to observe what an awesome dancer he was.

Neither I nor my husband James, ever told Darrington that he was included in our Will, but since he didn't live to reap the benefits, we have decided to arrange for a $25,000.00 Scholarship Memorial in his name by way of Albion Community Foundation and also a $10,000.00 Scholarship by way of Battle Creek Community Foundation. Per his request, the scholarships will focus on three areas, which all were of the utmost importance to him. Foremost it will benefit those who want to further their education in the area of Physical Therapy and who have maintained at least a 3.5 grade point average even though he maintained a 3.8. He was very specific about the grade point average as he wanted to be sure that only the serious applicants received assistance.

Darrington had worked hard to obtain such high marks and he always seemed to love a good educational challenge as well. He was proud of himself for having such stellar performance. The second area of focus will address the health needs of the impoverished who live in Calhoun County, such as: transportation to/from doctor appointments, financial assistance for the purpose of purchasing medications, health education programs, etc. Last, it will support educational programs that focus on issues relating to LGBTQ, Lesbian, Gay, Bisexual, Transgender and also those who are in Question.

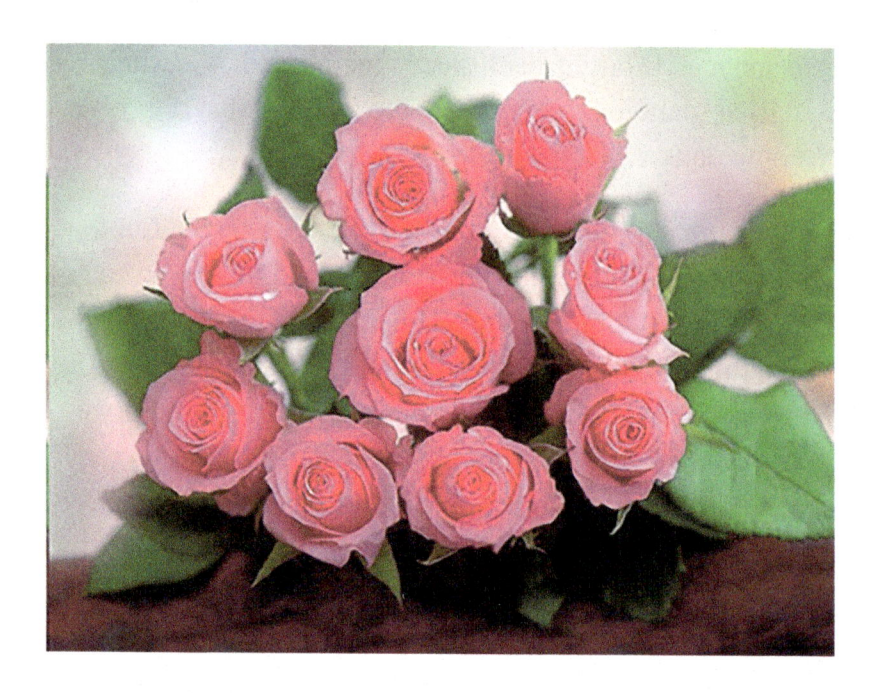

Especially for my dad, mom and sisters Jaquita and Barongiere

I don't want anyone to cry and grieve for me, for now I'm free!

I followed the plan God laid for me.

I've seen both grandpas and finally met Great Grandma Madeline too

Mom, I very clearly heard God's call, so

I took His hand and left it all...

Dad, I just could not stay another day, Not even to dance, to work or play;

Tasks left undone must stay that way.

Bari, for sure my parting has left you a huge void,

But promise me you'll fill it with remembered joy.

A friendship shared, a kiss and a choreographed Mime dance perchance even a Ballroom dance with you too.

Ah yes, for sure, these things too I will miss!

Oh Mom, my life's been very short but full, and I've savored So much, Good times, good family and friends, a loved-one's touch

Jaquita, I'm sure you think my time was all too brief but

Please don't shorten yours with undue grief.

Dad, it makes no sense to be burdened with tears of sorrow.

I pray that you enjoy the sunshine of the morrow

Even though I'm physically gone, spiritually I'm with you and I see you clearly... it is amazing...I can see twice as much as I could before. Sshh, can't you hear it...the sound of heaven is calling my name! All I see is beauty... copious, absolutely marvelous! I have to go now.

All My Love, your son and brother,
Darrington L.E.

Brothers and sisters, we do not want you to be uninformed about those who sleep in death, so that you do not grieve like the rest of mankind, who have no hope. For we believe that Jesus died and rose again, and so we believe that God will bring with Jesus those who have fallen asleep in him. According to the Lord's word, we tell you that we who are still alive, who are left until the coming of the Lord, will certainly not precede those who have fallen asleep. For the Lord himself will come down from heaven, with a loud command, with the voice of the archangel and with the trumpet call of God, and the dead in Christ will rise first. After that, we who are still alive and are left will be caught up together with them in the clouds to meet the Lord in the air. And so we will be with the Lord forever. Therefore, encourage one another with these words.
- 1 Thessalonians 4:13-18

May the blessings of the Lord be upon you my dear ones

REMEMBERING DARRINGTON

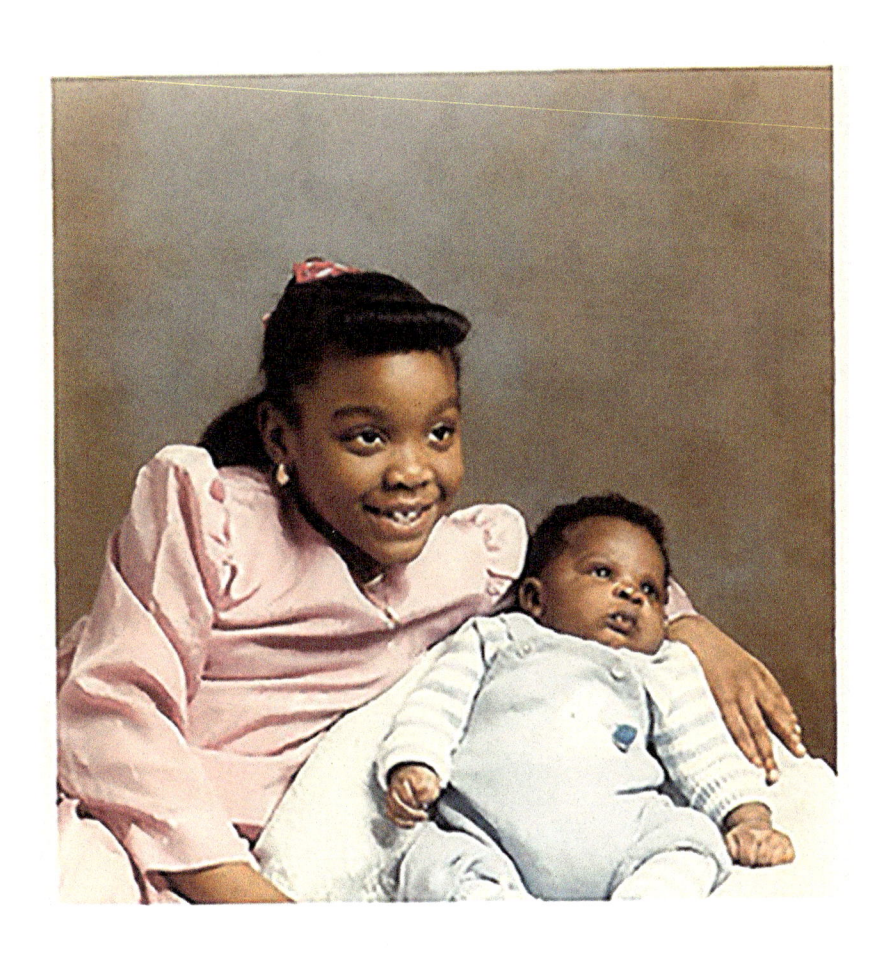

Destiny Fulfilled

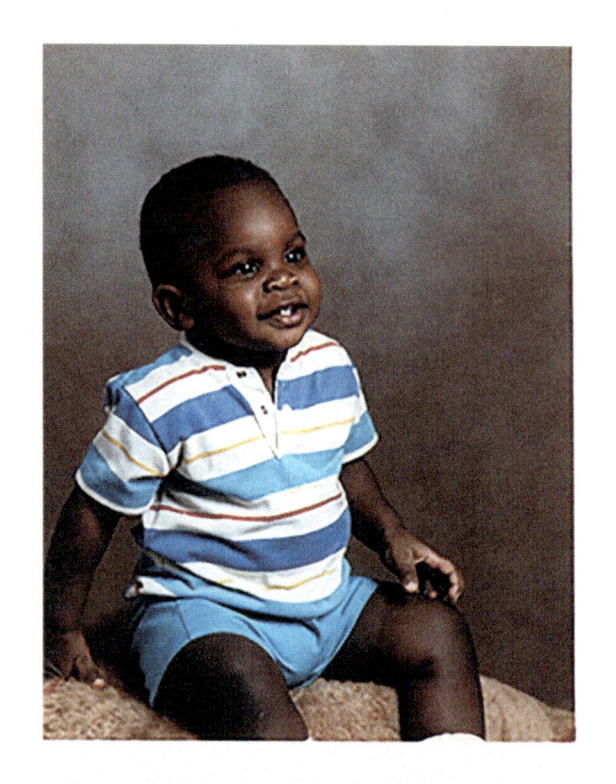

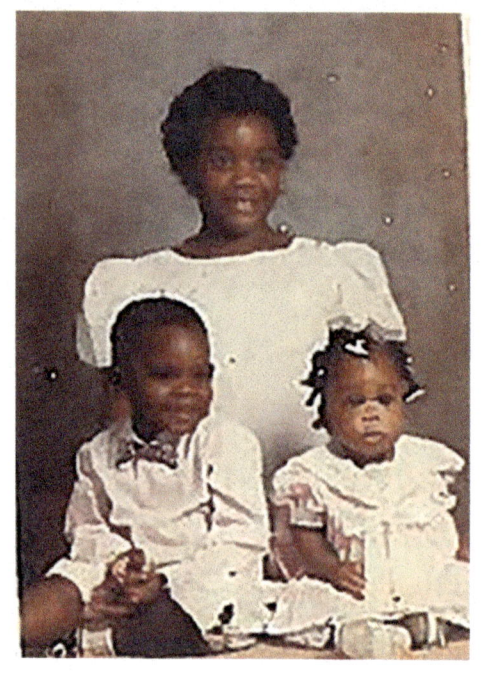

Remembering Darrington

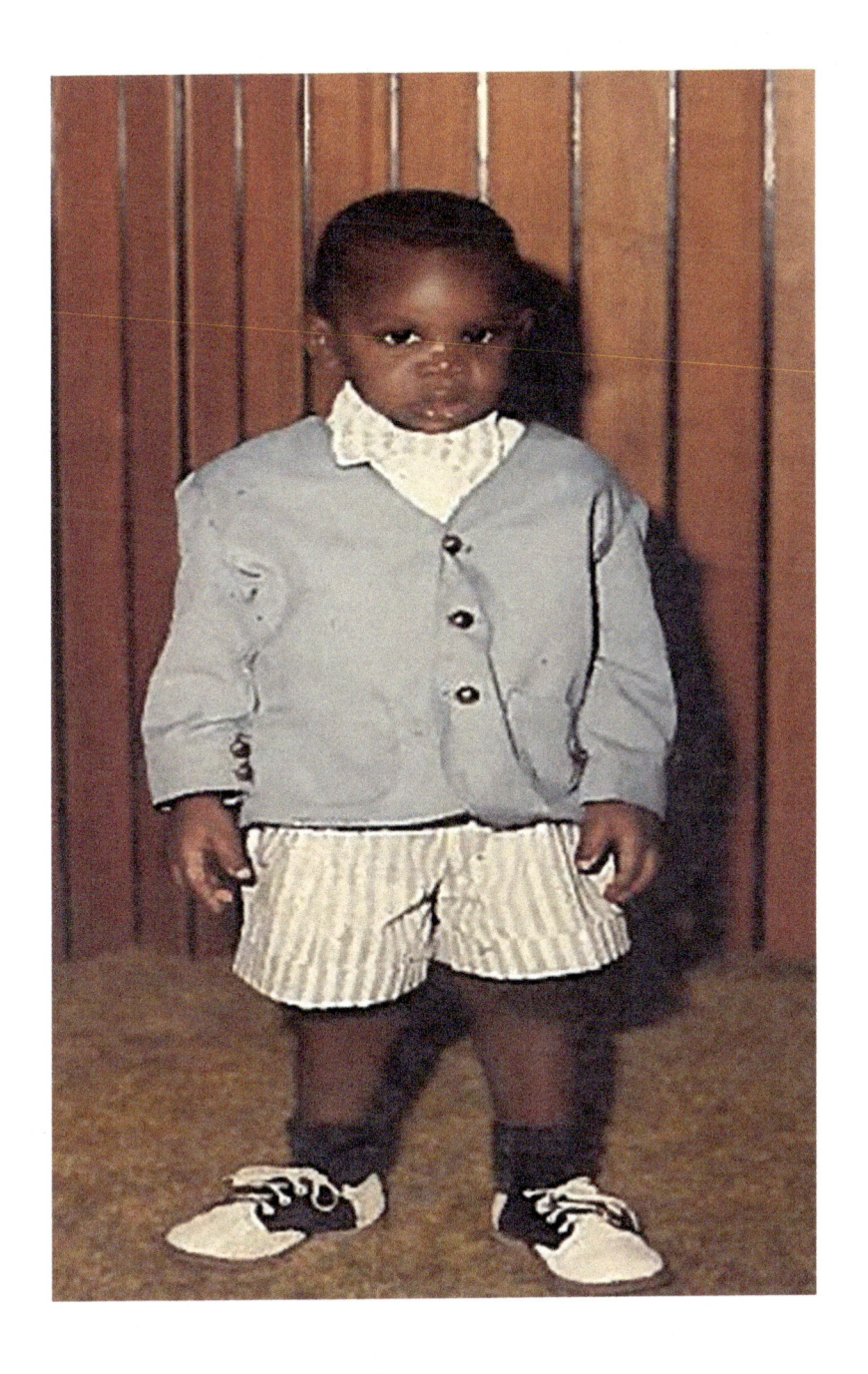

Destiny Fulfilled

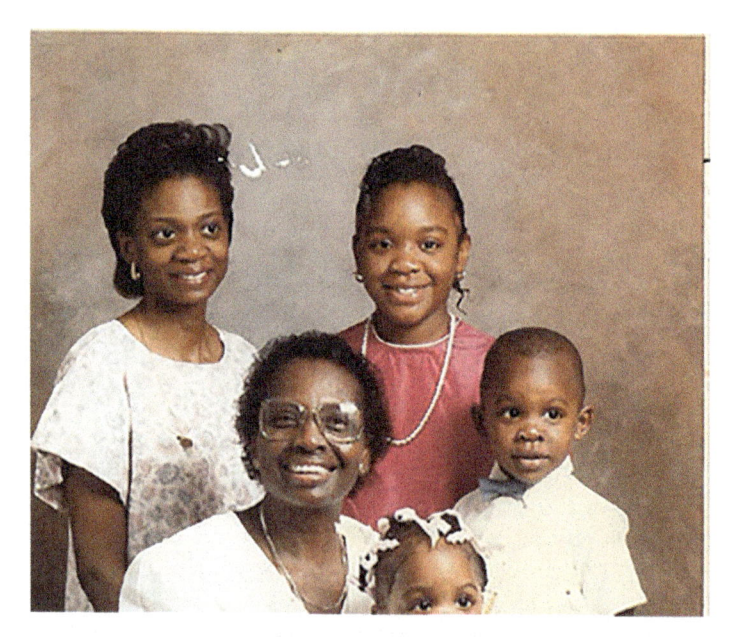

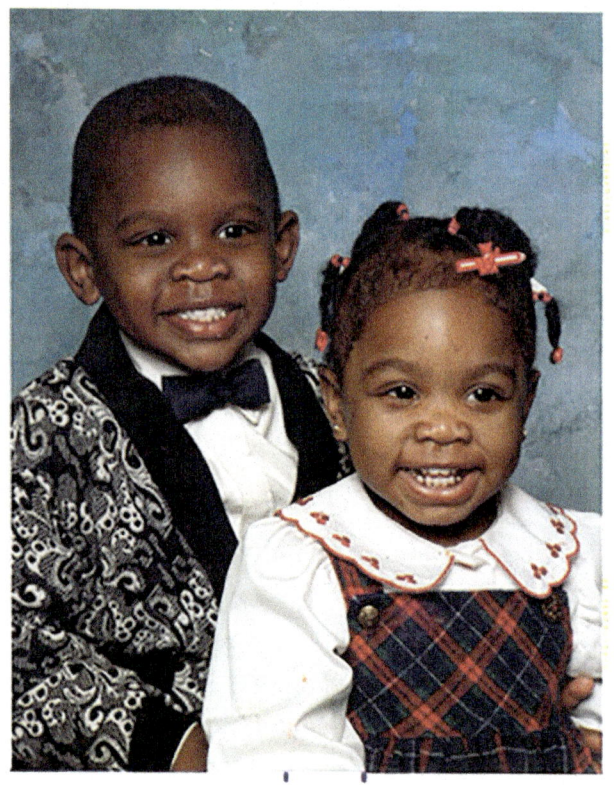

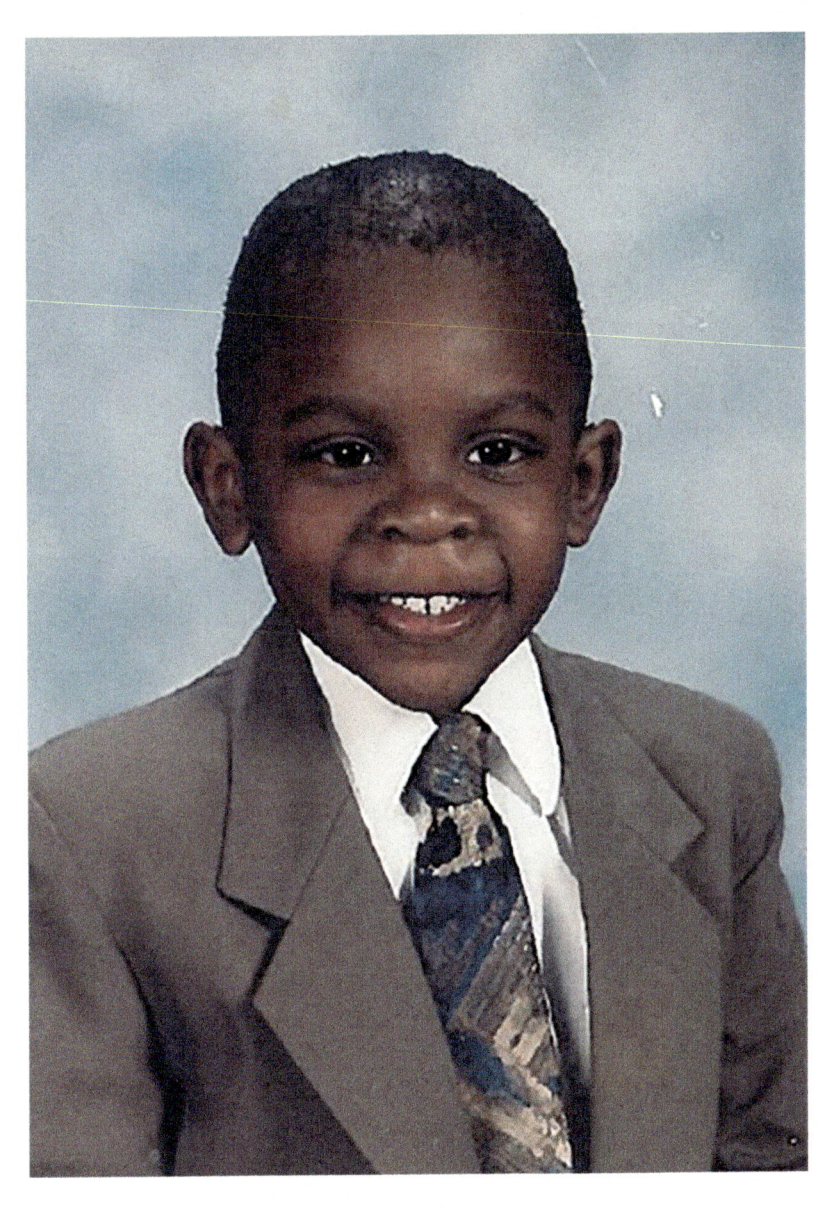

Love others the way that God has loved you, with tenderness.

— **Mother Teresa**

Destiny Fulfilled

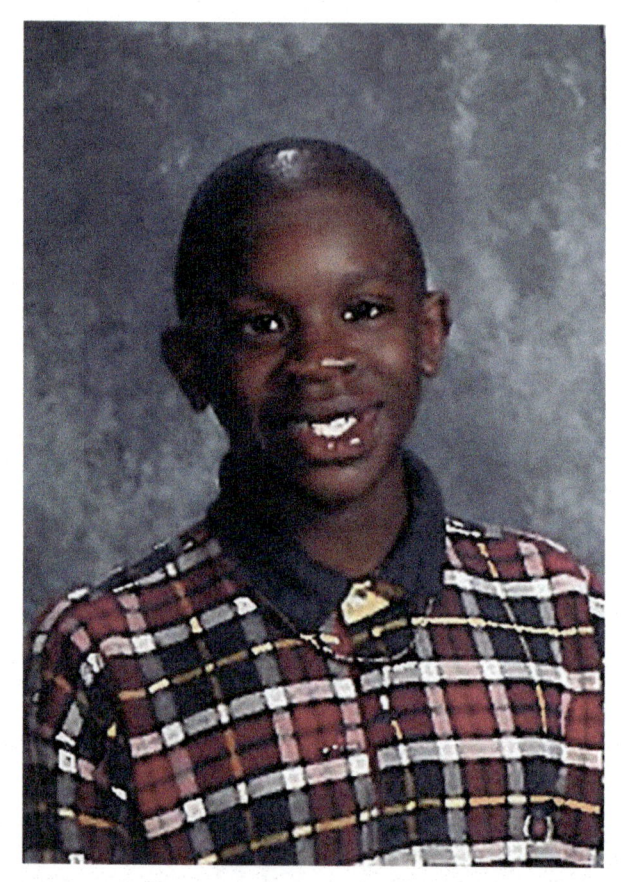

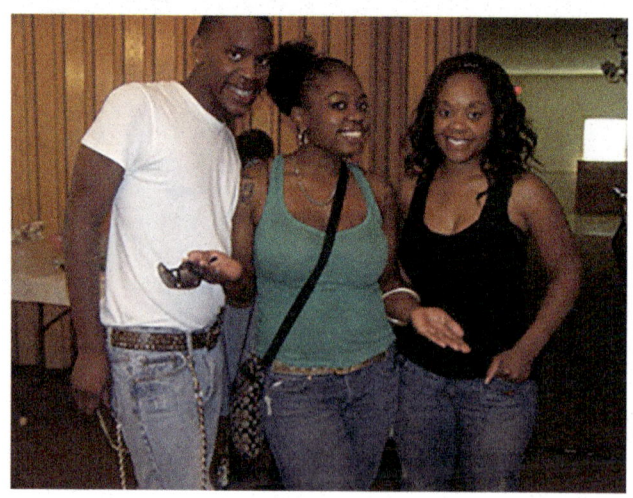

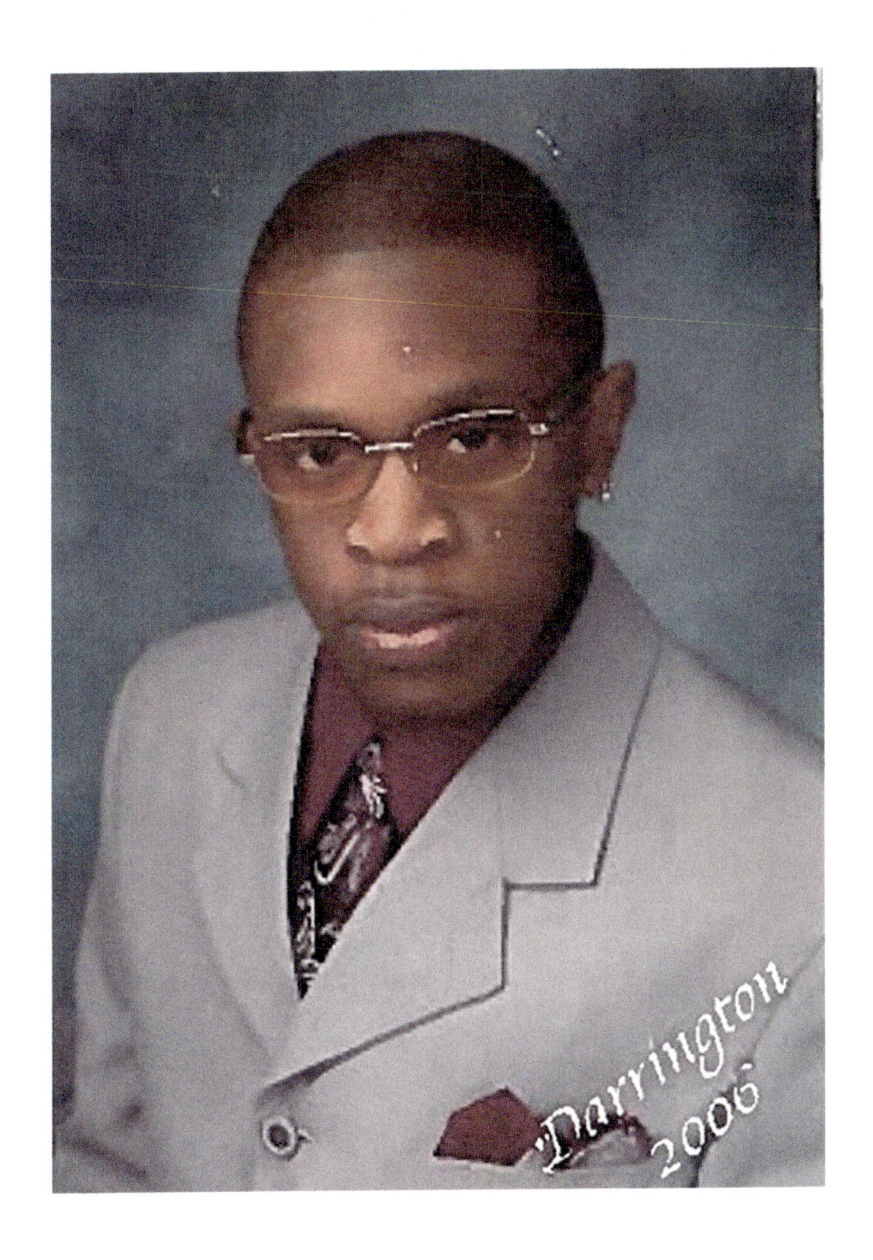

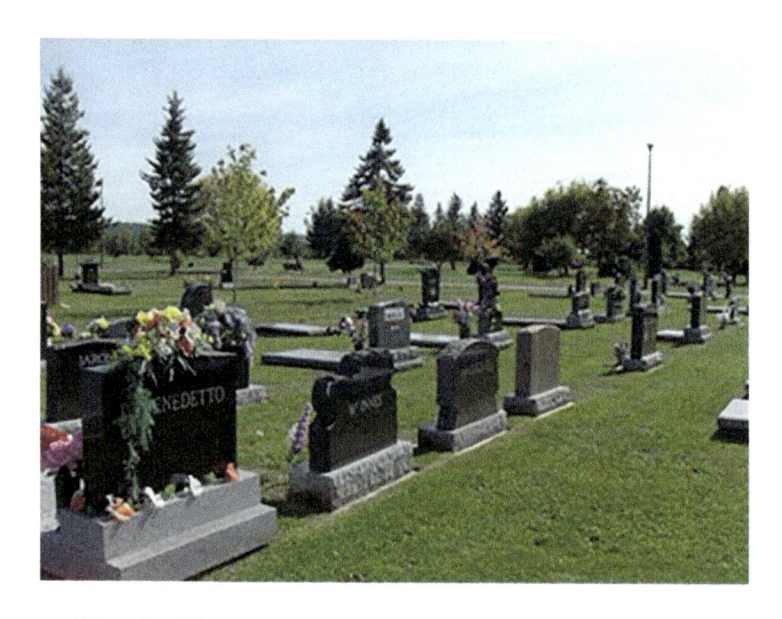

"Earth Has No Sorrow That Heaven Cannot Heal"

~**Martin Luther King Jr.**~

PART TWO:

DIET & HEALTH RESEARCH

CHAPTER TWELVE

LIL BIT OF WISDOM

Throughout my twenty-six years of working in the health field, I've certainly seen my share of illnesses and the damage that it does to the mind, body and soul. I am not naive, certainly there are some illnesses that are caused by genetics and no matter how many precautions are taken, it will not change the outcome. The more educated I become I find that many illnesses have more to do with diet and less with genetics. Basically when I speak to the average patient about the most minuscule diet change, versus the possibility of improved health, they look at me as if I'm incredulous.

Our generation has been programmed to believe that we must have surgery and a pill in order to fix our ailments. The thought of a simple diet change as a regiment to heal the body never crosses their mind and is totally unacceptable. If we don't change our way of thinking, there will be no hope for the younger generation and they will suffer the same or worse health issues than us. Mama always said, "Everybody got a lil bit of wisdom, and everybody got a lil bit of sense" Sometimes I'm not sure if either is true, but that is no excuse to do nothing. A Dietician once told me, "Always listen to your body, it will tell you what it wants and what it doesn't". I know that many of our illnesses have been brewing for years and we have chosen not to listen. Too often we choose to ignore the small aches, intermittent pains, and bothersome twinges.

We must now choose to become better listeners to our bodies

and stop assuming that good health habits are only for the wealthy. We must now choose to educate ourselves and not leave our health in the hands of our doctors or even the government. We must accept that doctors are trained to treat symptoms, not to investigate the root cause of our symptoms. Sadly, they have not been trained to look at the effect that our diet has on our body. I know this to be true because I've had the opportunity to speak to a number of them who were doing their residency. We must know more about our bodies than the doctors. Perhaps we may require surgery and a pill, but first let us exhaust our own theories that involve proper diet and exercise. It has been my experience that my doctors have not only appreciated but also welcomed my thoughts and ideas regarding my body. The information that we provide to our doctors will serve as a baseline from which to begin our treatment and will save us both a lot of frustration, time, effort, and most of all, our money. When we get to this point, then and only then will we be considered as sagacious.

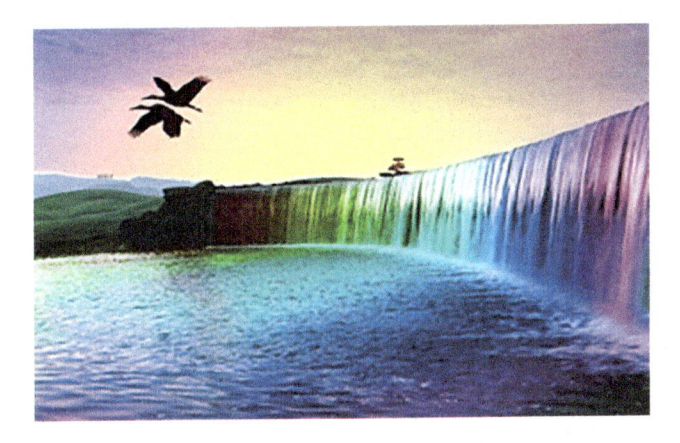

It is for us to make the effort. The result is always in God's hands.
       -Mahatma Gandhi, Indian political leader

CHAPTER THIRTEEN
CANCER FACTS

Blessed are those who find wisdom, those who gain understanding, for she is more profitable than silver and yields better returns than gold.
Proverbs 3:13-14 New International Version (NIV)

Research

In 1903, Thomas Edison predicted that "the doctor of the future will give no medicine, but instead will interest his patient in the care of the human frame, diet and in the cause and prevention of disease." A hundred and one years later, the American College of Lifestyle Medicine was born. According to Dr. Michael Gregor, Author of "How Not to Die", indicates that lifestyle docs still prescribe meds when necessary, but, based on the understanding that the leading causes of disability and death in the United States are caused mostly by lifestyle, our emphasis is particularly on what we put in our mouths: food and cigarettes. Several studies have shown that our lifestyles are the cause of many of our health problems, but the good news is that by changing our lifestyle we can dramatically improve our health.

As of 1950 research indicates that Japan's Colon Cancer was rated less than 1/5 of that of the United States, which also accounts for Americans of Japanese Ancestry. At this time the rate of colon cancer in Japan is equal to that of the United States which is mainly attributed to the diet and most likely focuses on meat consumption. In the past, studies have been done on both humans and animals, specifically on identical twins and on honeybees as well. Even though twins have the exact genes, it is possible that one could be healthy and the other, terminally ill based on how they each lived and what they experienced during their lifetime.

Epigenetics now deals with the control of gene activity. The skin cells are very different from bone cells, brain cells, and heart cells; but yet they all have the same complement of DNA. The end result is they each have different genes turned on or off. The queen bee and worker bees are genetically identical, but yet the queen bees store up to two thousand eggs a day and the worker bees are sterile. Queens can live up to three years while the workers may live only three weeks. The only difference between the two is diet. When the hive's queen is dying, a larva is picked by nurse bees to be fed a secreted substance called allied royal jelly. After the larva eats the jelly, the enzyme that had been silencing the expression of royal genes is turned off, and consequently a new queen bee is born. The queen has the exact same genes as any of the workers, but because of what she ate, different genes are expressed, and her life and the life span are significantly altered as a result.

Dr. Gregor's findings indicate that Cancer cells can use Epigenetics to turn off tumor suppressor genes that could otherwise halt the cancer. Dr. Gregor further states that even if you're born with good genes, cancer can find a way to turn them off. There are many Chemotherapy drugs that have been developed to help our body restore our natural defenses, but they're limited, due to high toxicity. I felt that because Darrington became so sick as a result of some of the medications, that he did experience some toxicity. It was very interesting to find that there are some plants that have the same natural effect such as: greens, beans and berries. One example includes dripping green tea on the colon, esophageal, or prostate cancer cells has been proven to reactivate genes silenced by the cancer.

What if we ate a diet chock-full of plant foods? In the Gene Expression Modulation by Intervention with Nutrition and Lifestyle (GEMINAL) study, Dr. David Ornish and colleagues took biopsies from men with prostate cancer before and after three months of intensive lifestyle changes that included a whole food plant based diet. Without any chemotherapy or radiation, beneficial changes in gene expression for five hundred different genes were noted. Within just a few months, the expression of disease preventing genes was boosted, and oncogenes that promote breast and prostate cancer were suppressed.

According to Dr. Greger, Americans lose more than five million years of life from cancers each year. A very small percentage are genetic, the remainder are caused by the environment, diet, etc. There are three cancers located within the digestive tract that claim one hundred thousand lives every year: colorectal (colon), pancreatic and esophageal.

Colorectal cancer is the second leading cause of cancer related death in the United States, yet in some parts of the world, it's unheard of. Colorectal cancer claims approximately 55,000 lives yearly, but is the easiest to cure if caught in time. 46,000 deaths are claimed from Pancreatic cancer each year; most don't live beyond the first year of

Cancer Facts

diagnosis. Eighteen thousand deaths are claimed from Esophageal cancer each year. Unfortunately, Pancreatic and Esophageal cancers which effect the tube between the mouth and the stomach are much more difficult to cure and are practically known as death sentences. Some foods that cause acid reflux directly affect the lining of the digestive tract and will have a direct impact on the esophagus.

More than one million people in the United States have been diagnosed with colorectal cancer before it spreads to the colon. There is about a 90 percent survival rate. Beginning at age 50–75 you should get stool testing every year and colonoscopies every ten years, according to Dr. Gregor.

Dr. Gregor has done extensive research in India and has found that India's gross domestic product (GDP) is approximately eight times less that than of the United States and approximately twenty percent of the people live in poverty. Women in the United States have up to ten times more Colorectal cancer than those in India. The women in the United States suffer seventeen times more lung cancer, nine times more endometrial and melanoma, twelve times more kidney cancer, eight times more bladder cancer and five times more breast cancer. Men in the United States appear to have eleven times more colorectal cancer than men in India, twenty-three times more prostate cancer, fourteen times more melanoma, nine times more kidney cancer and seven times more lung and bladder cancer than the people of India.

The large discrepancy may be explained by the regular use of a spice Turmeric used in Indian cooking. India is one of the world's largest producers of fruit and vegetables. Only seven percent of the Indian population eats meat on a regular basis. Actually only very little of the turmeric is absorbed into the blood stream and what doesn't go into the blood stream, goes directly into the colon to the cells that line your large intestine where cancerous polyps develop. Only about seven percent of the Indian population eats meat on a daily basis, the rest consume a diet of dark green, leafy vegetables and legumes, such as beans, split peas, chickpeas, and lentils, all which are packed with cancer fighting compounds called phytates. The regular use of the spice turmeric in Indian cooking has been proposed as a possible explanation. Curcumin, which is a yellow pigment in the spice turmeric, may be effective against cancer cells in vitro. Very little curcumin that you eat is absorbed into the bloodstream, so it may never actually come in contact with tumors outside the digestive tract. On the other hand, that which doesn't get absorbed in the blood ends up in your colon where it could impact the cells lining your large intestine where cancerous polyps develop according to Dr. Gregor.

Dr. Gregor's clinical findings indicate that Colon cancer is basically divided into three stages: aberrant crypt foci (abnormal clusters of cells along the lining of the colon. Second the polyps that grow from the inner surface the benign polyp transforms into a cancerous one. Last, when a benign polyp transforms itself into a cancerous one. Studies have shown that smokers in the first stage who have consumed cur- cumin for six months have shown a 40 percent decrease in cancer associated structures in the rectum within thirty days. In those where the polyps had already developed, after six months' use of curcumin along with quercetin which is naturally found in fruit and vegetables were shown to decrease the number of polyps by half in those with a hereditary form. In those that were in the very advanced stages and had failed chemotherapy and radiation, the oncologist started them on turmeric extract. In two of the four month treatments, the turmeric appeared to stall one third of the patients.

Phytates

Dr. Gregor's research also notes that Colorectal cancer is the second leading cause of cancer related death in the United States yet in some parts of the world it is practically unheard of. The highest rates have been recorded in Connecticut and the lowest in Kampala Uganda. Why is Colon Cancer so much more prevalent in the Western cultures? Renowned surgeon Denis Burkitt spent twenty-four years in Uganda. Many of the Ugandan hospitals that Dr. Burkitt visited had never even seen a case of colon cancer. He eventually came to the conclusion that fiber intake was the key as most Ugandans consumed diets centered around whole plant foods.

Subsequent research has suggested that dietary prevention of cancer may involve something other than just fiber. For instance, colorectal cancer rates are higher in Denmark than in Finland, yet Danes consume slightly more dietary fiber than Finns. Other research suggested that dietary prevention of cancer may involve something other than just fiber. For instance, colorectal cancer rates are higher in Denmark. Fiber isn't the only thing found in whole plant foods that is missing from processed and animal based foods according to Dr. Gregor and his extensive medical research.

It's possible that the answer lies in natural compounds, called phytates which are found in seeds of plants: whole grains, beans, nuts and seeds. Phytates have been shown to detoxify excess iron in the body which otherwise can generate a particularly harmful kind of free radical called hydroxyl radicals. Meat contains the type of iron particularly associated with colorectal cancer but lacks, as do refined plant foods, the phytates to extinguish those iron forged free radicals. Those who eat foods high in phytates are known to have less bone loss, and fewer hip fractures. Dr. Gregor states that there was a six-year study done in California which concluded that the higher the meat consumption, the higher risk of colon cancer.

Unexpectedly white meat was worse. Those who ate red meat at least once each week had about double the risk of developing colon cancer, the risk tripled for those who ate chicken or fish once or more a week. Eating beans was found to help mediate some of that risk so your colon risk may be determined by your meat to vegetable ratio. It may not be enough to cut down on your meat, but also you may need to eat more plants. The National Cancer Institute Polyp Prevention Trial found that those who increased their bean consumption by even less than one quarter cup a day appeared to cut their odds of precancerous colorectal poly recurrence by up to 65 percent based on the research of Dr. Gregor.

Phytates are credited with reduced risks because they are known to inhibit the growth of virtually all human cancer cells tested so far including cancers of the colon breast cervix, prostate, liver, pancreas, and skin while leaving normal cells alone.

Dr. Gregor indicates that Phytates target cancer cells through a combination of antioxidant, anti-inflammatory and immune enhancing activities. Besides affecting the cancer cells directly, phytates have been found to boost the activity of natural killer cells, which are white blood cells that form your first line of defense by hunting down and disposing of cancer cells. Phytates can also play a role in your last line of defense which involves starving tumors of their blood supply. There are many photo nutrients in plant foods that can help block the formation of new blood vessels that feed tumors, but phytates also appear able to disrupt sting tumor supply lines. Similarly, many plant compounds appear able to help and slow down and even stop cancer cell growth, but phytates can sometimes also cause cancer cells to apparently revert back to their normal state, which would be to stop behaving like cancer cells as well as in cancer cells of the breast, liver and prostate.

Stool Size Matters

Dr. Gregor indicates that the larger and more frequent the bowel movements, the healthier you may be. Based on a study of twenty-three populations across a dozen countries, the incidence of colon cancer appears to skyrocket as the averse daily stool weight drops below about a half a pound. Populations dropping quarter pounders have three times the rate of colon cancer. You can actually measure your stool by weighing yourself before and after you expel it. The link between stool size, and colon cancer may be related to the amount of time it takes for the stool to travel through the colon. The larger the stool, the quicker the transit time. Wow! People fail to realize that you can actually have a bowel movement and still be constipated, which people find very difficult to believe.

Gregor notes that even if you're eating a plant based diet, it generally takes one or two days to be digested by a man that eats a plant based diet, but about five days if he eats a conventional diet. Women will expel a plant based meal in about a day or two, but four days if it's conventional. If it takes less than twenty-four to thirty-six hours, you're probably right on target. Constipation is the most common gastrointestinal complaint in the United States.

Colon cancer rates increase when the weight of the stool is less than a half pound. Of course straining to pass small firm stools also play a role in causing many health problems, including hiatal hernias, varicose veins, hemorrhoids, and painful conditions such as anal fissure. Constipation can also be considered a nutrient deficient disease and that nutrient is fiber. You can get constipated if you don't consume enough fiber. Since fiber is found only in plant foods, it stands to reason that the more plants you eat, the less likely you are to be constipated according to Dr. Gregor.

Too much iron

Dr. Gregor's findings indicate that during the year 2012, the results from two major Harvard University studies were published. The first, known as the Nurses' Health Study, began following the diet of about 120,000 women aged thirty to 55 starting back in 1976; the second, the Health Professional Follow up study, followed about 50,000 men aged 40-75. Every four years, researchers checked in with study participants to keep track of their diets. By 2008 a total of about 24,000 subjects had died including 6000 from heart attack and 9,000 from cancer.

The researchers found that the consumption of both processed and unprocessed red meat was associated with an increased risk of dying from cancer and heart disease and shortened life span overall. They concluded that even after controlling for age, weight, alcohol consumption, exercise, smoking, etc. The findings suggested that the subjects weren't dying early because they ate less of some beneficial compound like phytate in plants, but instead that there may have been something harmful in the meat itself. The largest study of diet and health in history is the NIH-AARP study, cosponsored by the National Institute of Health and the American Association of Retired Persons.

Over the course of a decade, researchers followed about 545,000 men and women aged 50 to 71 in the largest study of meat and mortality ever conducted. The scientists came to the same conclusion as the Harvard researchers: Meat consumption was associated with increased risk of dying from cancer, dying from heart disease and dying prematurely in general. This was determined after controlling for other diet and lifestyle factors, effectively excluding the possibility that people who ate meat also smoked more, exercised less, or failed to eat their fruits and veggies. The accompanying editorial in the American Medical Association's Archives of Internal Medicine (titled "Reducing Meat Consumption Has Multiple benefits for the World's Health) called for a major reduction in total meat intake.

Dr. Gregor believes that Heme iron which is contained in meat can generate cancer causing free radicals by acting as pro oxidant, iron can be considered a double-edged sword; too little of it and you can risk anemia, too much may increase risk of cancer and heart disease. The body naturally tries to balance the amount of iron in the system. Once you have sufficient amount of iron in the system the body is five times more effective at blocking the absorption of excess iron from plant foods than from animal foods.

This may be why Heme iron is associated with cancer and heart disease risk according to Dr. Gregor. Similarly, Heme iron is associated with higher risk of diabetes, but Non Heme iron is not. If we remove iron from people's bodies, can we decrease cancer rates? Studies have found that people randomized to give regular blood donations to reduce their iron stores appear to cut their risk of getting and dying from new gut cancers by about half over a five-year period. The meat industry is working on coming up with additives that suppress the toxic effects of Heme iron, but a better strategy may be to emphasize plant source in your diet, which your body can better manage.

Gregor's research further indicates that vegetarians who eat a plant based diet actually consume more iron than those who don't because the iron is not absorbed into the system as efficiently as the Heme iron in meat. Also women who eat plant based diets do not appear to have iron deficiencies more than women who eat lots of meat.

Pancreatic Cancer

Dr. Gregor states that Pancreatic Cancer is known for its aggressiveness and for being the most lethal of cancers. Unfortunately, there hasn't been a lot of definitive research done. The NIH-AARP conducted a large enough study to be able to tease out what kind of fat was most associated with it. It was the first to separate out the role of fats from plant sources, such as those found in nuts, seeds, avocado and olive and vegetable oils, versus all animal sources, including meats, dairy products and eggs. The consumption of fat from all animal sources was significantly associated with pancreatic cancer risk, but no correlation was found with the consumption of plant fats.

The recent study of 30,000 poultry workers, was diagnosed specifically to test whether exposure to poultry cancer-causing viruses that widely occurs occupationally in poultry workers-not to mention the general population-may be associated with increased risks of deaths from liver and pancreatic cancers. The study found that those who slaughter chicken have about nine times the odds of both pancreatic cancer and liver cancer. To put this result in context, the most carefully studied risk factor for pancreatic cancer is cigarette smoking, but even if you smoke for fifty years, you'd have only doubled your odds of getting pancreatic cancer. Regarding the people who actually ate chicken, researchers found a 72 percent increased risk of pancreatic cancer for every fifty grams of chicken consumed daily, which is just under two ounces.

Curcumin appears able to reverse precancerous changes in colon cancer and has been shown in laboratory studies to be effective against lung cancer cells. In a study funded by the National Cancer Institute and performed at the MD Anderson Cancer Center, patients with advanced pancreatic cancer were given large doses of curcumin. Of the 21 patients the researchers were able to evaluate, two responded positively to the treatment. One had a 73 percent reduction in his tumor size, though eventually a curcumin resistant tumor developed in its place. The other patient showed steady improvement unless curcumin breaks occurred. Until more research has been done, follow a plant-based diet, avoid smoking, tobacco and added sugars per Dr. Gregor.

Esophageal Cancer

According to Dr. Gregor, the tube that carries food from the mouth to the stomach is the esophagus. Each year, eighteen thousand people are diagnosed with the disease and approximately fifteen thousand lives are claimed by it. Primary risk factors include: smoking, alcohol drinking (even mild to moderate) and esophageal reflux (GERD). When the acid from the stomach, goes up the throat and causes a burning sensation, it destroys the lining of the esophageal and causes cancer. Besides avoiding tobacco, the most important thing to do is avoid the acid reflux through diet. Fat intake is associated with increased acid reflux and fiber appears to decrease it. A high fiber intake may reduce the incidence of esophageal cancer by as much as 1/3 by helping to prevent the root cause of many cases of acid reflux: the herniation of part of the stomach up into the chest cavity. Within five minutes of eating fat, your sphincter muscle at the top of your stomach (which keeps food down) relaxes and allows acids to enter back into your esophagus. This may be due to a release of a hormone called cholecystokinin, which is triggered by both meat and eggs and may also relax the sphincter. This may also explain why those who eat meat have been found to have twice the odds of reflux induced to esophageal inflammation compared with vegetarians. The best way to manage this may be to avoid the foods that allow acids to escape. The most protective foods are: orange, red, and dark green leafy vegetables, berries, apples, citrus fruits, but all unprocessed plant foods have the advantage of high fiber.

Dr. Gregor determines that the increased abdominal pressure may also back up blood flow in the veins around the anus, causing hemorrhoids, and even push blood flow back into the legs resulting in varicose veins. But a fiber rich diet can relieve the pressure in both directions. Those who eat plant food diets that revolve around whole plant foods tend to pass such effortless bowel movements that their stomachs stay where they're supposed to, which can reduce acid spillover implicated in one of our deadliest cancers. If you aren't constantly filling your bowels with plant foods, the only natural source of fiber, unwanted waste products can get reabsorbed and undermine your body's attempts at detoxifying itself. Only three percent of Americans may even reach the recommended minimum daily intake of fiber, making it one of the most widespread nutrient deficiencies in the United States.

Dr. Gregor's findings indicate that researchers have tested strawberries as a possible cure for Esophageal Cancer. In a randomized clinical trial of powdered strawberries in patients with precancerous lesions in their esophagus, subjects ate one to two ounces of freeze-dried strawberries every day for six months-that's the daily equivalent of about a pound of fresh strawberries. All of the study participants started out with either mild or moderate precancerous disease; but amazingly, the progression of the disease was reversed in about eighty percent of the patients in the high dose strawberry group. Most of these precancerous lesions either regressed from moderate to mild, or disappeared entirely. Half of those on the high dose strawberry treatment walked away disease free.

Yvonne Thomson, Health Coach, has a wealth of knowledge about health in general. Yvonne credits her own mother, Norma Amburgey for teaching her infinite health advantages of a proper diet, vitamins, supplements, etc. as a child. She has passed the baton onto her children and grandchildren as well.

Her clinical findings indicate that good health begins in the gut. In contrast, an unhealthy gut is the beginning of most, if not all, physical and mental disease. The key to a healthy gut requires perfect balance of gut flora, or bacteria. Environmental toxins, vaccinations, antibiotics, prescription drugs, stress, lack of sleep, and poor eating habits all affect that delicate balance. Thomson has worked with many clients who have had joint pain, mental fogginess, obesity, sluggishness, and those who strongly want to improve their overall health, gut health should be the primary focus. By focusing primarily on the gut, she has been able to assist many clients bring their body back into balance.

CHAPTER FOURTEEN
EXERCISE

Jessica Kellner, *Mother Earth Living* editor in chief, also an Exercise Enthusiast, states that exercise is crucial to our health, both physical and mental-in so many ways that whether we hope to shed a few pounds is irrelevant to whether we should commit to a daily exercise program. Exercise's most commonly noted health effects often center on our cardiovascular systems; Exercise is key to maintaining heart health; reducing risk factors of heart disease; and reducing risk of death from heart disease (as well as all other causes of mortality). But it also yields many additional benefits. Some 90 percent of Americans don't get enough exercise. In fact, researchers believe many of the declines we consider a natural part of aging may well be as much from lack of use as from the march of time. Kellner shares how exercise effects many aspects of the mind and body.

CANCER PREVENTION: Kellner research indicates that when it comes to cancer prevention, exercise is highly effective at reducing risk-especially against certain forms of cancer. The key, however is in the level of intensity: Those who exercise vigorously see a significantly higher protective effect than those who exercise at low intensity. In one study, researchers monitored more than 2,500 middle-aged Finnish men for about 17 years, documenting daily activity levels. After controlling for cigarette smoking, fiber and fat intake, age and other variables, the scientists concluded that the most physically active men were the least likely to develop cancer, in particular of the gastrointestinal tract or lungs. But according to reporting by The New York Times, the intensity of the activity was key, those who jogged or did similarly intense exercise for at least 30 minutes a day had a 50 percent reduction in the risk of dying prematurely of cancer while those who stilled and walked saw smaller reductions in risk. Quantity is also important: In the comprehensive 2008 national Physical Activity Guidelines Advisory Committee report, the committee found that one hour per day of moderate vigorous activity reduced risk of breast cancer more significantly than the 2.5 hours of moderate exercise a week recommended by the surgeon general.

IMMUNITY: Exercise reduces incidents of cold, flu and infection. Based on a study of about 1,000 healthy adults aged 18-85 over a 12-week period, those in the top quarter for fitness level (who exercised five days a week) experienced 43 percent fewer days with upper respiratory tract illness compared with the bottom 25 percent of exercisers. Exactly why exercise may boost immunity is a mystery. Some researchers hypothesize that exercise helps increase the diversity of the beneficial microorganisms in the gut, thereby improving the immunity. Studies have linked exercise with greater diversity in the microbiota. Some believe the immune benefits may be connected with exercise's positive effects on circulation, while others attribute the increase in wellness to the reduction in stress hormones exercise confers. One caveat: After intense, extended workouts (runs of more than two hours, for example) immune function is temporarily diminished.

BONE HEALTH: When we are young exercise helps build strong bones and achieve greater peak mass which continues throughout our twenties more so than those who don't. Based on studies from the National Institute of Arthritis and Musculoskeletal and Skin Diseases, following that time period, we begin to lose bone every year; but exercise can help to prevent bone loss. Not all exercise boosts bone health, however-exercises such as cycling and swimming while excellent cardiovascular exercises, don't help protect the bones because they're not weight bearing. Instead, try exercises that make the body work against gravity: weight training, hiking and jogging, tennis, dancing or climbing stairs.

JOINT AND BACK PAIN: Exercise strengthens joints, which can reduce the effects of the degenerative disease osteoarthritis. Although it may seem counterintuitive, exercise helps increase joint flexibility and health. Many arthritis patients who start an exercise program report less disability and pain, and also remain independent longer than their inactive peers, according to research reported in The New York Times. Some of the best exercises for osteoarthritis sufferers include strengthening exercises such as weight lifting; range-of motion exercises such as yoga and tai chi; and low impact aerobics such as swimming, cycling and walking. Lack of exercise may also increase risk of low back pain for those with chronic pain. Some of the best exercises to maintain strength and flexibility in the back include yoga and tai chi, low impact aerobic exercise, and the development of strong core muscles. Those with chronic low back pain should be guided by professionals, however, as strenuous activity can also exacerbate back pain.

BALANCE: Every year, more than a third of seniors age 65 or older fall and these falls can have serious health impacts when they lead to fractures or concussions. Balancing exercises are important to help maintain health, and they can also make us more agile and thus less prone to injury during other types of exercise. Balance is readily regained with practice and balancing exercises are easy to do at home.

MUSCLE LOSS: Some muscle loss is unavoidable. Beginning at age 30 we lose approximately one percent of muscle every year, but researchers say that we can significantly slow this process with weight training. A 70-year-old active individual is probably younger from a biomarker standpoint-muscle strength, balance, body composite, blood pressure, cholesterol levels than a 40-year-old inactive individual, Miriam Nelson, a professor of nutrition at Tufts University, told the Boston Globe. She found in studies that previously sedentary postmenopausal women could increase muscle strength by 80 percent by lifting weights twice a week for a year. Beginning middle age, everyone should aim to do twice weekly, strength training, weight lifting or body weight bearing exercises such as push-ups squats and lunges. In order to build muscle, we need to consume protein. According to an article published in The Boston Globe, research states that seniors may need nearly double that in order to avoid accelerated muscle (46 grams for women and 56 for men) loss. Total amount of protein should not be consumed all at once; but instead, most should be eaten in the morning and the rest throughout the day.

ANXIETY AND DEPRESSION: Kellner's research extends into the mental health areas as well. Both Anxiety and Depression are among the most common mental illnesses. Depression affects 25 percent of Americans at some point in their lives. Anxiety disorders affect another 18 percent of Americans. Prescription drugs are the most common treatment-use of prescription antidepressants increased by 400 percent between 1988 and 2008 according to the Centers for Disease Control and Prevention, and more than one in 10 Americans older than twelve takes an antidepressant. Yet multiple studies have found exercise to be just as effective as pharmaceuticals in treating the symptoms of depression and anxiety. A 1999 randomized controlled trial found that an aerobic exercise program improved symptoms in depressed adults as much as the drug Zoloft, reports The Atlantic. A 2006 meta-analysis of 11 studies backed up these findings. Researchers have also found exercise to positively impact the pathophysiological process of anxiety, with numerous studies and meta-analysis finding exercise to be associated with reduced anxiety. Although researchers can be sure of all the ways exercise benefits those with these disorders, one recent study suggests that exercise may calm neurons in the brain. Researchers have known that exercise can build new neurons. Often these new neurons are predisposed to be easily excited, firing wildly at the slightest provocation. However, exercise also creates new neurons specifically designed to release the brain calming neurotransmitter GABA. In essence, exercise helps the brain respond quickly to stress; but to calm down much more quickly after the stressful event, keep unnecessary anxiety at bay. Researchers say quantity and intensity are important. Most recommend 45-50 jute sessions three to five days a week, aiming to reach 50 to 80.5 percent of maximum heart rate.

MENTAL PERFORMANCE AND CONCENTRATION

According to Harvard Medical School, exercise can improve mental function including: memory, concentration and mental sharpness. Regular moderate intense workouts benefit the brain by maintaining healthy blood pressure, lifting mood and lowering stress, it also has a direct effect on brain chemicals. Exercise stimulates brain regions involved in memory to release a chemical called brain-derived neurotrophic factor (BDNF), according to Harvard Health Publications, the media division of Harvard Medical School. BDNF rewires memory circuits to work more effectively. "Not so long ago, neuroscientists assumed that humans were born with a certain number of brain cells-and that was it throughout one's life," according to Karen Postal, a neuropsychologist and clinical instructor at Harvard Medical School. "Now it's clear that new cells are born throughout our lives, in the area of the brain responsible for laying down new memories, and this process is triggered by exercise. When we exercise and it has to be enough to really sweat neurogenesis, or the birth of new cells is the result." And, while exercise is how we generate new cells we must put them to work in order for them to stick around. So consider taking a run, then following it up with a crossword puzzle, by practicing a new language or instrument or by cooking an unfamiliar dish.

SLEEP: Exercise's relationship with sleep seems obvious: Fatigue in our bodies during the day helps us sleep better at night. And for those without sleep disorders, this is often the case. However, when using exercise to treat insomnia in formerly sedentary individuals, results might take a while. A clinical psychologist and sleep researcher at Northwestern

University, Kelly Glazer Baron, was fond of prescribing exercises for her patients with insomnia. However, she often heard them complain that it didn't help. Yet studies had shown exercise to be an effective treatment for the disorder. Digging into past studies, Baron discovered that because those with sleep disorders tend to have "what we characterize as a hyper arousal of the stress system," as she told The New York Times it takes longer for exercise to benefit their sleep. In fact, it can take as much as four months, long enough for exercise to help calm the underlying physiological arousal. Although results aren't immediate (and exercising consistently can be more difficult without adequate sleep) after four months the test subjects Baron examined were getting at least 45 minutes more sleep per night, which she says is as good or better than the most current treatment options including pharmaceutical drugs.

CHAPTER FIFTEEN
DIET & NUTRITION

Supplements

Kathie Madonna Swift, a registered Dietary Nurse, author of "The Swift Diet" and Education Director for Food as Medicine, a professional nutrition training program for physicians and other health care providers, states that, "Because each person's needs are different, supplementation can't be a one size fits all approach. Supplementation often requires the skill of a credentialed nutritionist or physician trained in integrative medicine," Swift says. The one supplement however, that Swift recommends for just about everyone is probiotics, which are so important for gut health. Look for a high quality, broad spectrum probiotic that contains a variety of Lactobacillus and Bifidobacteria strains. Swift suggests that people start with a dose of about 1 to 10 billion colony forming units (CFUs).

Foods -According to the American Journal of Epidemiology

Patients who follow a plant based diet have reduced mortality from all causes, but also a decreased risk for cancer overall. One study in particular, found that eating a whole foods diet is associated with a significantly lower risk for stomach cancer. Other research, published in the American Journal of Epidemiology, found that post-menopausal women who eat a plant-based Mediterranean diet had a reduced risk of breast cancer. Although all plant-based whole foods are good for the body, the foods that seem to be the oat protective against cancer include: Blueberries, Olive Oil, and Tomatoes.

Blueberries are untried and antioxidant powerhouses that have been linked to everything from reducing blood pressure to preventing cancer. They're rich in powerful antioxidant compounds that help protect the body and the body's DNA from damage from exposure to things such as pesticides, pollution and poor diet, all of which trigger the formation of disease forming molecules called free radicals.

A Spanish study of Olive Oil found that adding as little as 10 teaspoons of olive oil to our daily diet could help protect women against breast cancer. The researchers theorize that olive oil may mount a multi- pronged attack on cancer tumors, stunting their growth, and even protecting against potentially cancerous damage to DNA. What's more, compelling research found that Oleoscanthal, a powerful antioxidant found in extra virgin olive oil-has been shown to wipe out cancer cells in as little as 30 minutes.

Tomatoes are rich in lycopene (a powerful antioxidant) which researchers from Wayne State University School of Medicine found seems to protect against cancer-particularly breast, prostate and kidney cancers. Lycopene is a carotenoid, responsible for giving many fruits and vegetables, especially tomatoes, their red color. Eating tomatoes with a little bit of olive oil helps the lycopene to be better absorbed by the body.

Swift suggests that by putting the right foods into our bodies, our immune systems can do their jobs of boosting our overall wellness and resistance to illness and disease. "Our immune system is in our gut," says Kathie Madonna Swift. "What we eat, therefore, affects how are bodies fight illnesses and disease", Swift says. The Ancient Greek physician, Hippocrates coined the phrase "Let food by thy medicine and medicine be thy food." Our Society has gotten so far away from real food, it is time to get back to the basics without all the processed, packaged and artificial ingredients.

Support Digestive Health-According to the American Journal of Clinical Nutrition

Researchers have determined that adding healthy bacteria into our bodies throughout diet or supplements can help reduce gas and bloating and increase regularity. The foods that help support a health digestive system include:

ALMONDS: These nuts have been found to be a good source of prebiotics which is essentially food the beneficial microorganisms in the intestine need to thrive. These nuts are also rich in fiber, which helps prevent a number of conditions, including constipation, acid reflux, inflammatory bowel syndrome and diverticulitis.

SAUERKRAUT: Fermented cabbage (aka sauerkraut) is packed with beneficial Lactobacillus bacteria, as well as cancer fighting compounds such as sulforaphane. These beneficial bacteria take up residence in the intestinal tract, which aids in digestion. Studies have also shown that this strengthening of the gut and the immune system can help prevent cancer.

GINGER: This herb is widely used to treat nausea and stomach upset, as well as morning sickness and motion sickness. Ginger contains a natural chemical that's used as an ingredient in antacid, laxative and anti-gas medications. One study from the University of Michigan Medical School found ginger reduced inflammation in the colon (a precursor to colon cancer) within just a month.

Grab n Go

Eleanor Hughes, Freelance Writer and the Outreach Coordinator for the University of Arkansas for Medical Science, suggests that we eat when we're hungry and make mostly nutritious choices like veggies, fruits, lean proteins, and whole grains. We should exercise and balance the calories we take in with the calories we burn off. The concept is elementary, but unfortunately, healthy eating is anything but simple. We make food choices for many reasons besides hunger: cravings, boredom, celebration, loneliness, convenience and lack of time. We live in a very busy world, nothing is easy, it seems that everything is a hassle. We may not have control over many things, but we do have control over what we eat and what we feed our families and what we snack on. A healthy snack consists of complex carbs such as veggies, fruits, and whole grains, paired with lean protein, such as eggs, seeds, nuts, beans and dairy. Eleanor recommends that healthy foods be divided into two sections: quick fix and make ahead. Quick fix is anything that you can toss together in two minutes. Make ahead foods should be made in big batches on the weekend.

Quick Fix Snack

Easy Turkey Wrap

Apple slices and homemade honey mustard dress up this old classic. Apples are a seasonal way to add fiber, texture, vitamins and minerals. For a savory wrap, replace the sliced apple with a handful of halved cherry tomatoes. You can use a 100 percent whole grain tortilla to wrap your dressed up turkey or opt for a crunchy lettuce leaf with virtually no calories

Whole grain tortilla, lettuce leaf or both
3 slices turkey (about 2 ounces)
2 teaspoons honey mustard
1/4 cup sliced apple

Healthier Honey Mustard for Wrap
1/2 cup plain Greek yogurt
2 tablespoons yellow mustard
1 1/2 tablespoons raw local honey
1 tablespoon lemon juice

Lay turkey slices atop tortilla and/or lettuce leaf.
Spread honey mustard on turkey and top with apple slices.
Roll up and enjoy
Makes 1 wrap
Recipe adapted from mywholefoodlife.com

Make Ahead Snacks

When you have some extra time over the weekend, here are a few ideas for healthy snacks that take some work on the front end, but are able save time in the end.

Banana Oatmeal Walnut Cookies

This cookie recipe is shockingly simple. Vitamin rich with potassium and pectin (a soluble fiber) and naturally sweet bananas stand in here for the sugar.

    2 medium ripe bananas, mashed
    1 cup quick oats
    1/4 cup chopped walnuts

-Combine mashed bananas with oats in a mixing bowl, then fold in the nuts.
-Place tablespoon sized scoops on a baking sheet and bake for -15 minutes in a 350-degree oven. Makes about 10 cookies.

- Recipe adapted from skinnytaste.com

Baked Lemon Kale Chips

Kale is one of the healthiest vegetables on the planet. By eating one cup of chopped kale, you are getting 9 percent of your daily needs for calcium, 206 of your vitamin A, 134 percent of your vitamin C and 685 percent of your vitamin k needs. Kale provides all this plus copper, potassium, iron, manganese and phosphorus for only 33 calories per cup. These crunchy kale chips make an excellent snack by themselves, and also crumble into a tasty seasoning. Stir a handful of the chips into a half a cup of cottage cheese to make a delicious, protein rich dip for vegetables

1 large bunch fresh kale
2 tablespoons olive oil
Juice and zest of 1 lemon
1 to 2 teaspoons kosher salt
Few twists freshly ground black pepper
1 dash each cayenne and garlic powder (optional)

-Preheat oven to 324 degrees.

-Trim thick stems out of kale. Chop remaining strips into bit size pieces.

-In a mixing bowl, stir together oil, lemon juice zest and seasonings. Toss kale in mixture and marinate for at least 30 minutes.

-Spread out marinated kale in a single layer on a baking sheet and bake for about 15 minutes or until edges begin to brown. -Let cool and store in an airtight container.

- Recipe by Tabitha Alterman.

So Much Better Than Deli Chicken

3-4 lb. whole chicken
3-4 T. extra virgin olive oil
2 garlic cloves, finely chopped
2-3 T. fresh herbs, finely chopped (Choose from your favorites. I like a mixture of rosemary, thyme, marjoram, sage, parsley, etc.)
Salt
Pepper

-Preheat oven to 500 degrees.

-Lightly grease a roasting pan or baking dish. Lay the chicken, breast side up, in the pan.

-In a small bowl combine the olive oil, garlic, mixed herbs, salt and pepper.

- Using hands, rub oil/herb mixture on the outside of the skin, underneath the skin (gently separating skin from meat with your fingers), and inside the cavity. After one side is done, flip bird over and do the same, using all the mixture. Leave the chicken breast side down for roasting.
- Place chicken, uncovered, in preheated oven. Set timer for 15 minutes.

Skin should show some browning. This will sear the outside so the meat will stay moist.

- Turn oven down to 300 degrees and continue to roast for approximately 1 1/2 hours, or until a meat thermometer inserted into the thickest part of the meat registers 160 degrees.
- Remove chicken from oven and tent with parchment paper to rest and keep warm until serving.

- Recipe by Yvonne Thomson, Health Coach

Roasted Asparagus

1-2 pounds fresh asparagus
Extra virgin olive oil
Salt

- Preheat oven to 425 degrees.
- Rinse asparagus thoroughly. Cut off and discard the coarse ends.
- Lay asparagus, in single layer on a baking sheet, lined with parchment paper. Drizzle olive oil over asparagus, being careful to cover each spear. Lightly, sprinkle salt over asparagus.
- Roast for 10 minutes.
- Serve immediately.

- Recipe by Yvonne Thomson, Health Coach

My people are destroyed from lack of knowledge. A people without understanding will come to ruin

- Hosea 4:6, 14

CONCLUSION

For certain we all lack knowledge and understanding to a certain degree, but since we know this to be true, let us vow to diligently pursue health and wellness education in hopes of obtaining a much higher level of knowledge and wisdom that cannot only help us, but our generation as a whole. History does not have to repeat itself. Based upon my research, knowledge and God-given wisdom, I've learned that 97 percent of our illnesses are caused by diet and a lack of exercise, and only 3 percent is actually caused by genetics. Let us move forward and not be ill advised by continuing to recite "I will eat and do whatever I want because something is going to kill me anyway."

Yes, we all will die someday, and yes the Coroner will assign us all a cause of death, which will no doubt be written on a pretty pink post it note that will probably dangle from our big toe. Following the Coroner's evaluation, a Mortician will be contacted to clean and cover up whatever messes we've made during our lifetime, before dressing us up to look absolutely fabulous for the funeral! Hopefully those visits will be a long way away, but until such time arrives, I think we should take every opportunity to obtain as much knowledge and understanding by first humbling ourselves, listening to our bodies, reading food labels, pay attention to what we're putting into our bodies, get some type of physical exercise daily, etc.

I am extremely offended when I hear the remarks of others about my nephew, "Girl, now you know Darrington was gonna die anyway." I definitely have some issues with these types of comments, especially when I know they specifically come from an ignorant point of view rather than factual research, case studies. You see I'm convinced that his cancer was in the making and his genes were very slowly going awry for many years prior to the date of diagnosis. With all my heart, I believe that the red flags were flying high and the signs and symptoms of his cancer were apparent when he was a small child, but our family had no idea what we were seeing. Last, I believe that even though we are all destined to leave this old world, the crucial information that we don't have and or what we don't know can be extremely detrimental to us. By choosing not to pursue this essential information, we can indeed expedite our time here on this side of heaven; and as an end result, we cannot blame our fate on either God or the Devil.

Based upon the latest scientific research, our happiness has a lot to do with our current health issues. Happiness has nothing to do with the amount of money we have in the back, and or our social status; however, it does determine how content we are with ourselves. Since we know that money cannot buy us love, good health and happiness, we need to look within ourselves and try to be happy rather than gloomy. Being happy could very well be the answer to reducing the amount of medicine that we take and or cancelling the surgery that we are scheduled to undergo.

Studies have shown that there is a significant difference between the average American and a happy individual. Research also suggests some helpful habits that we should adopt in order to at least try to increase our level of happiness.

Conclusion

First, we need to be social by reaching out to others; ***Darrington knew no strangers; he always wanted to acquaint himself with others***. Second, spend wisely, prioritize your health, unplug from our electrical devices at least once in a while, go outside, practice gratitude, laugh, spend time with happy people, be altruistic, sleep well, don't be on the negative, and just let go emotionally of things that we have no control and or the ability to change. *As a last resort we could all do as Darrington did and "dance our ass off." Though he passed away at a young age, it really worked wonders for him emotionally.*

It is my opinion that both men and women alike, feel that if they dwell on their problem long enough it will somehow magically disappear…. poof. No, our problems don't dissipate but it's quite possible that you will end up in either one of two predicaments: counseling for depression/anxiety and or surgery. I've seen it over and over and over. A Pastor Elmer Hess said, "If you're going to worry, then don't pray, and if you're going to pray, why worry?" I realize that this is easier said than done, but we must try. We must remember that happiness is a choice and we can choose to be happy just as easily as we can choose to be miserable.

More than anything that I've mentioned, we should never forget that we only have today, as tomorrow is not promised to any of us. It is an honor to be on God's "wake up" list, because not everyone will be. We don't want to go through life only to find that we have wasted what could have been a beautiful experience by worrying about something that we had absolutely no control over. I don't think we realize how much unfavorable energy we bring into our lives that actually cause stress and consequently leads to mental and physical illnesses.

Also, I find that we put too much negative energy into being jealous and envious of each other. What I see on a regular basis is that there are many people who are very humble, work hard and delay gratification; while some chose to do nothing at all, but yet put a lot of negative energy into being jealous of others who have accomplished what field they would have actually liked to. We have to remember that nothing of any great value will ever come without a lot of hard work, effort, and a fair amount of disappointments.

Darrington was desperate to roll up his sleeves and work hard to earn his education and Lord knows he had his share of disappointments. He wasn't walking around hoping that he would somehow magically acquire it, nor did he sit and make a lot of adverse comments about those who had already obtained it. I have worked with the public for the last twenty-six years and I have not only heard it all, but seen it all as well.

At this point, I feel that my life is 50/50 meaning that 50 percent of my success and or my health will be based upon my attitude and the remaining 50 percent will be based upon the choices that I make. When someone tells me "no," right away, I then say to myself, "but why not," and or "maybe you're right, but let's just give it a try anyway." You see, I intend to defy the odds of the expectations of pessimists and I will continuously strive to obtain as much information as possible to keep myself healthy and sagacious, as I won't let my nephew's death be in vain. Will you join me?

Conclusion

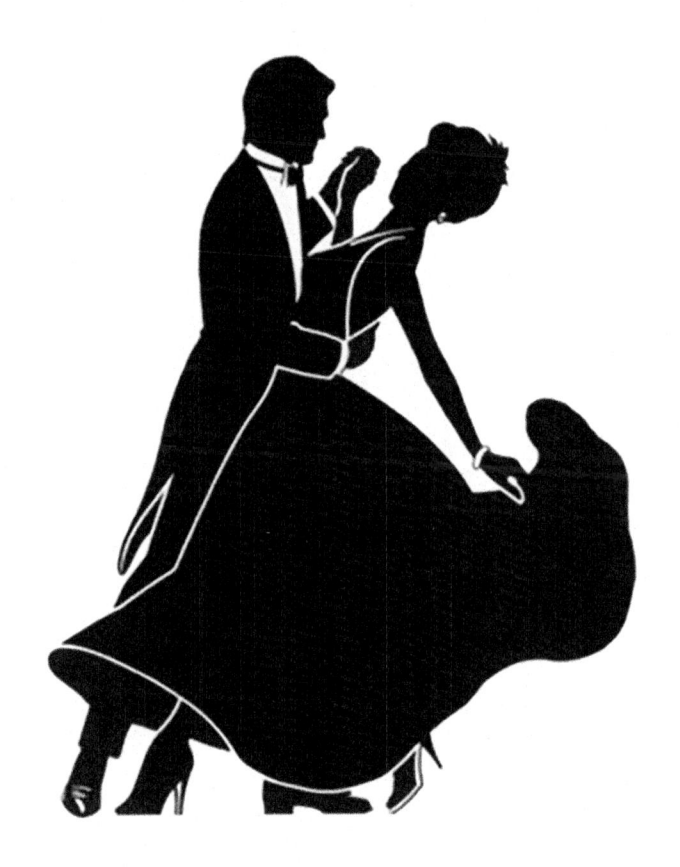

Hey Shelly, I see Lori at the bar, let's go say hello and get ourselves a nice cold drink of water and perhaps a small lettuce salad.

Okay Darrington, that sounds like a wonderful idea, but first you've got to show me some of those smooth dance moves that you make look so easy!

The End

INDEX

Quotes:

Page 1   Matthew 5:4 Holy Bible-New Living Translation

Page ix   Sirach 6:14-16 Revised Standard Version Catholic Edition Island & irish.com/page/folks/bless.html

Page xi   Romans 5:2-5 New International Version

Page 4   1 John 3:14

Page 8   Romans 8:38-39

Page 9   Mathew 6:9-13

Page 21   Psalm 146:2

Page 22   Ecclesiastics 3:4

Page 23   Proverbs 4 King James Version

Page 39   Jeremiah 10:12 New International Version

Page 39   Reverend James Cleveland

Page 41,137   Pastor Elmer Hess Sr

Page 41   Robin Williams, Actor

Page 42,78,97   Mother Teresa, Albanian Roman Catholic Nun And Missionary

Page 42   Prince Rogers Nelson, Singer, Song writer, Actor

Page 42   Psalm 139:14

Page 46   2 Chronicles 7:4

Page 55   1 John 3:18

Page 63   John 3:16

Page 70   Leo Sullivan, darn good friend!

Page 78   Mother Teresa

Page 80   Alfred Lord Tennyson, British Poet

Page 80   Deuteronomy 32:39

Page 84   2 Timothy 4:7

Page 92   1 Thessalonians 4:13-18

Page 97   Mother Teresa

Page 100 Martin Luther King Jr, Theologian, Civil Rights

Page 103 Mahatma Gandhi, Indian Political Leader

Page 104 Proverbs 3:13-14

Page 104 Thomas Edison, Inventor & Businessman

Page 104 Dr. Michael Gregor, Author of How Not to Die

Page 118 Yvonne Thomson, Health Coach

Page 119 Jessica Kellner, Mother Earth News Guide to, Edi Natural Health/Summer 2016 Chief/ Summer 2016

Page 126, 128   Kathie Madonna Swift, Registered Dietary Nurse, Author of the Swift Diet, Mother Earth Living/Summer 2016

Page 129 Eleanor Hughes, Freelance Writer & Outreach Coordinator for the University of Arkansas for Medical Sciences. Mother Earth News Guide to Natural Health/Summer 2016

Page 133 Yvonne Thomson

Page 134 Hosea 4:6,14

Page 137 Pastor Elmer Hess Sr

ABOUT THE AUTHOR

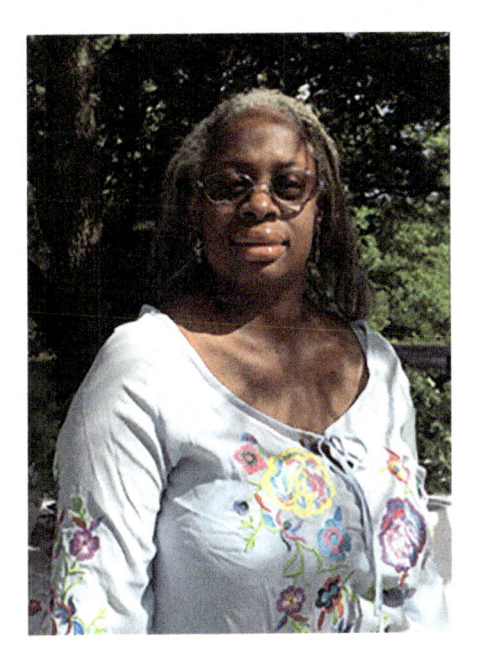

Gladys Seedorf was born in 1963 in Cambridge Maryland. She has a Master's Degree and 25 years' experience in the Home Health Care and Hospice field. Currently she is working towards a doctoral degree in Philosophy of Psychology.

Gladys lives with her husband in Battle Creek, Michigan. She is also the author of **What Mama Said**, and **Bittersweet**.